LICK THE SUGAR HABIT SUGAR COUNTER

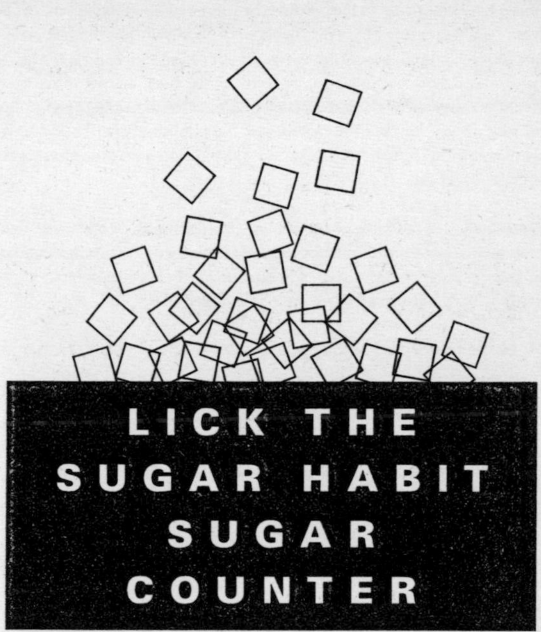

LICK THE SUGAR HABIT SUGAR COUNTER

Discover the Hidden Sugar in Your Food

Nancy Appleton, Ph.D.

AVERY a member of PENGUIN PUTNAM INC.

New York

Every effort has been made to ensure that the information contained in this book is complete and accurate. However, neither the publisher nor the author is engaged in rendering professional advice or services to the individual reader. The ideas, procedures, and suggestions contained in this book are not intended as a substitute for consulting with your physician. All matters regarding health require medical supervision. Neither the author nor the publisher shall be liable or responsible for any loss, injury, or damage allegedly arising from any information or suggestion in this book.

Most Avery books are available at special quantity discounts for bulk purchase for sales promotions, premiums, fund-raising, and educational needs. Special books or book excerpts also can be created to fit specific needs. For details, write Putnam Special Markets, 375 Hudson Street, New York, NY 10014.

a member of
Penguin Putnam Inc.
375 Hudson Street
New York, NY 10014
www.penguinputnam.com

Published simultaneously in Canada

Library of Congress Cataloging-in-Publication Data

Appleton, Nancy.
Lick the sugar habit sugar counter : discover the hidden sugar in your food / Nancy Appleton.
p. cm.
Includes bibliographical references.
ISBN 1-58333-093-3
1. Food—Sugar content. I. Title.
TX553.S8 A67 2001 00-069994
613.2'83—dc21

Printed in the United States of America

10 9 8 7 6 5 4 3 2 1

BOOK DESIGN BY MAUNA EICHNER

Contents

Fast Foods 165

Introduction

Why I Wrote the *Lick the Sugar Habit Sugar Counter*

Fifteen years ago I wrote a book called *Lick the Sugar Habit*. Now in its fourth edition, the book is more relevant today than ever before. Despite the overwhelming evidence that excess sugar is hazardous to our health, the average American consumes as much as 153 pounds of added sugar per year. This is equivalent to over a half cup of sugar a day. The average teenage boy eats twice that much. I compiled this counter because I found that many people need to know how much sugar is in the food that they are eating. This book gives you that information quickly and easily. As I gathered the data for this book, I was startled to find out how much sugar is hidden in so many products. For example, did you know that sugar is added even to "salty" foods such as ketchup, breads, and crackers? Did you also know that sugar is often added to foods such as bacon, salt, pastrami and other processed luncheon meats, sushi, roasted nuts, spaghetti sauce, frozen dinners, bouillon cubes, and non-dairy creamer? There are various reasons why sugar is used in products that do not seem to need it: Some manufacturers believe that sugar is a necessary ingredient in products made with yeast, such as bagels; sugar is sometimes used by manufacturers as an inexpensive filler; and manufacturers know that sugar makes their products tastier, which keeps consumers coming back for more.

Here is another bit of interesting information. When I lecture, I ask the audience if they know how many grams there are in one teaspoon of sugar. Literally no one knows—no one. And yet on each package that you buy in a grocery store, the grams of sugar are listed, not the teaspoons. I know very few people who think in terms of grams, and the result is that the consumer has no useful understanding of how much sugar is in a product. Let me enlighten you. **There are approximately 4 grams of sugar in every teaspoon of sugar.** Now you can start calculating how many teaspoons of sugar you eat each day. You will be amazed.

The Negative Effects of Sugar on the Body

Can you go for more than a day without eating sugar in any form? Do you drink soft drinks or milkshakes, eat Danish pastries, fruit yogurt (a 6-ounce serving has seven teaspoons of sugar or honey!), donuts, bagels, cakes, cookies, muffins, or other sugary items? Can you forgo foods that contain ingredients with words ending in "ose" such as sucrose or fructose, or contain corn syrup, corn sweetener, honey, barley malt, maple syrup, sugar-cane solids, or rice syrup? Do you frequently indulge in a carton of ice cream or on a bag of cookies? If you find that these sugary items are part of your everyday diet, you may have a problem. You may say, "Who cares? What's wrong with sugar?"

There is significant scientific evidence written in many medical journals showing that sugar can ruin your health. (See "110 Reasons Why Sugar and Sweeteners Are Ruining Your Health" on pages 5–14.) Do you have any of the following symptoms? Do you feel sleepy after meals, have allergies, gas, bloating, extended stomach after meals, joint pains, headaches, chronic fatigue, constipation, diarrhea, excess weight, skin problems, or high blood pressure? These all can be signs of a sugar problem.

In order to understand why eliminating sugar from your diet is beneficial, you must understand how sugar is processed by your body. Our early ancestors ate foods high in fiber and nutrients containing natural sugars in limited amounts. Today we eat a diet of highly refined, processed foods, many of which are full of fats and sugars. Our digestive systems are not equipped to digest this glut of high-sugar, nutrient-poor foods.

Researchers are now discovering what happens to the minerals in the body when sugar and other abusive foods, such as fried food and over-processed foods, are eaten. For example, every time we eat just as little as two teaspoons of sugar, our blood chemistry can change, throwing our bodies out of balance (out of homeostasis). Sugar upsets the balance of minerals in the body and can change their relationship to one another. (Minerals only work in relation to one another.) In the presence of excess sugar, calcium increases while phosphorus decreases, upsetting the optimal ratio. In this case, calcium becomes toxic in the body and can cause plaque on the teeth, kidney stones, arthritis, cataracts, bone spurs, hardening of the arteries, gallbladder stones, and other problems.

When mineral levels decrease dramatically, our enzyme function can be impaired, because enzymes, too, are dependent upon minerals to perform properly. As a result, we may not digest our food completely, and some of this partially digested food can get directly into the bloodstream where it is treated as a foreign substance. The medical community is now calling this condition *leaky gut syndrome* or *gut permeability*. This byproduct of incomplete digestion is a form of food allergy. It forces the immune system to respond and, for many of us, results in respiratory ailments (sneezes and wheezes) and inflammation. For others it might cause headaches, irritability, arthritis, fatigue, multiple sclerosis, psoriasis, or other problems.

In short, too much sugar overworks, exhausts, and weakens our immune system. It plays havoc with the endocrine system, depleting some hormones and causing an imbalance in body chemistry. The white blood cells, triggered by the immune system to fight disease, need protein to function. If they do not receive the correct protein combinations, due to incomplete digestion, the immune system cannot function properly. Again, this constant immune system response eventually exhausts the body, and once the immune system becomes suppressed, the door is opened to innumerable infectious and degenerative diseases.

For a more complete understanding of what sugar does to the body, read my book *Lick the Sugar Habit.* This book also contains recipes (some delicious and sweet without sugar, fruit, or fruit juice), food plans, techniques to overcome sugar addiction, and much more.

110 Reasons Why Sugar Is Ruining Your Health

You might want to copy this list and put it on your refrigerator or tape it to your sugar bowl!

1. Sugar can suppress the immune system.
2. Sugar upsets the balance of minerals in the body.
3. Sugar can cause hyperactivity, anxiety, difficulty concentrating, and crankiness in children.
4. Sugar can produce a significant rise in triglycerides.
5. Sugar contributes to a reduction of defense against bacterial infection.
6. Sugar causes a loss of tissue elasticity and function.
7. Sugar reduces high density lipoproteins.
8. Sugar leads to chromium deficiency.
9. Sugar leads to cancer of the breast, ovaries, prostate, and rectum.
10. Sugar can increase fasting levels of glucose.
11. Sugar causes copper deficiency.
12. Sugar interferes with the absorption of calcium and magnesium.
13. Sugar can weaken eyesight.

14. Sugar raises the level of the neurotransmitters dopamine, serotonin, and norepinephrine.
15. Sugar can cause hypoglycemia.
16. Sugar can produce an acidic digestive track.
17. Sugar can cause a rapid rise of adrenaline levels in children.
18. Sugar malabsorption is frequent in patients with functional bowel disease.
19. Sugar can cause aging.
20. Sugar can lead to alcoholism.
21. Sugar can cause tooth decay.
22. Sugar contributes to obesity.
23. High intake of sugar increases the risk of ulcerative colitis.
24. Sugar can cause changes frequently found in people with gastric or duodenal ulcers, including inflammation and destruction of the digestive tract, acute hunger, and pain after eating or while lying down.
25. Sugar can cause arthritis.
26. Sugar can cause asthma.

27. Sugar can cause *Candida albicans* (yeast infections).
28. Sugar can cause gallstones.
29. Sugar can cause ischemic heart disease.
30. Sugar can cause appendicitis.
31. Sugar can cause multiple sclerosis.
32. Sugar can cause hemorrhoids.
33. Sugar can cause varicose veins.
34. Sugar can elevate glucose and insulin responses in oral contraceptive users.
35. Sugar can lead to periodontal disease.
36. Sugar can contribute to osteoporosis.
37. Sugar contributes to saliva acidity.
38. Sugar can cause a decrease in insulin sensitivity.
39. Sugar leads to decreased glucose tolerance.
40. Sugar can decrease growth hormone.
41. Sugar can increase cholesterol.
42. Sugar can increase the systolic blood pressure.

43. Sugar can cause drowsiness and decreased activity in children.

44. Sugar can cause migraine headaches.

45. Sugar can interfere with the absorption of protein.

46. Sugar causes food allergies.

47. Sugar can contribute to diabetes.

48. Sugar can cause toxemia during pregnancy.

49. Sugar can contribute to eczema in children.

50. Sugar can cause cardiovascular disease.

51. Sugar can impair the structure of DNA.

52. Sugar can change the structure of protein.

53. Sugar can make our skin age by changing the structure of collagen.

54. Sugar can cause cataracts.

55. Sugar can cause emphysema.

56. Sugar can cause atherosclerosis.

57. Sugar can promote an elevation of low density proteins (LDL).

58. Sugar can cause free radicals in the bloodstream.

59. Sugar lowers the enzymes' ability to function.

60. Sugar can permanently alter the way proteins act in the body.

61. Sugar can increase the size of the liver by causing liver cells to divide.

62. Sugar can increase the amount of liver fat.

63. Sugar can increase kidney size and produce pathological changes in the kidney.

64. Sugar can damage the pancreas.

65. Sugar can increase fluid retention.

66. Sugar is the number one enemy of bowel movement.

67. Sugar can cause myopia (nearsightedness).

68. Sugar can compromise the lining of the capillaries.

69. Sugar can make the tendons more brittle.

70. Sugar can cause headaches.

71. Sugar can over-stress the pancreas.
72. Sugar can adversely affect school children's grades.
73. Sugar can cause an increase in delta, alpha, and theta brain waves.
74. Sugar can cause depression.
75. Sugar increases the risk of gastric cancer.
76. Sugar can cause dyspepsia (indigestion).
77. Sugar can increase the risk of gout.
78. The ingestion of sugar can increase the levels of glucose in an oral glucose tolerance test over the ingestion of complex carbohydrates.
79. Sugar can increase the insulin response in those who consume high-sugar diets compared to those who consume low-sugar diets.
80. Sugar increases bacterial fermentation in the colon.
81. Sugar can cause less effective functioning of two blood proteins, albumin and lipoproteins, which may reduce the body's ability to handle fat and cholesterol.

82. There is a greater risk for Crohn's disease with people who have a high intake of sugar.
83. Sugar can cause platelet adhesiveness.
84. Sugar can cause hormonal imbalance.
85. Sugar can lead to the formation of kidney stones.
86. Sugar can lead to the hypothalamus becoming highly sensitive to a large variety of stimuli.
87. Sugar can lead to dizziness.
88. High-sugar diets significantly increase serum insulin.
89. High-sugar diets of subjects with peripheral vascular disease significantly increases platelet adhesion.
90. High-sugar diets can lead to biliary tract cancer.
91. High-sugar diets tend to be lower in antioxidant micronutrients.
92. High-sugar consumption of pregnant adolescents is associated with a twofold increased risk for delivering a small-for-gestational-age (SGA) infant.

93. High sugar consumption can lead to substantial decrease in gestation duration among adolescents with high-sugar diets.
94. Sugar slows food's travel time through the gastrointestinal tract.
95. Sugar increases the concentration of bile acids in stools and bacterial enzymes in the colon. This can modify bile to produce cancer-causing compounds and colon cancer.
96. Diets high in sugar can increase fasting blood glucose.
97. Sugar combines and destroys phosphatase, an enzyme, which makes the process of digestion more difficult.
98. Sugar can be a risk factor of gallbladder cancer.
99. Sugar is an addictive substance.
100. Sugar can be intoxicating, similar to alcohol.
101. Sugar can exacerbate premenstrual syndrome (PMS).
102. Sugar suppresses lymphocytes.

103. A decrease in sugar intake can increase emotional stability.

104. The body changes sugar into two to five times more fat in the bloodstream than it does starch.

105. The rapid absorption of glucose promotes excessive food intake in obese subjects.

106. Sugar can worsen the symptoms of children with attention deficit disorder (ADD).

107. Sugar adversely affects urinary electrolyte composition.

108. Sugar can slow down the functioning ability of the adrenal glands.

109. Sugar has the potential to induce abnormal metabolic processes in a normal healthy individual and to promote chronic degenerative diseases.

110. High-sugar intake could be an important risk factor in lung carcinogenesis.

For the sources for "110 Reasons Why Sugar Is Ruining Your Health," see pages 203–212.

Sugar in All Its Forms

Sugar comes in many forms and has many names. To help you identify sugar on product labels, here are some of sugar's aliases.

barley malt

beet sugar

brown sugar

cane sugar

cane syrup

cane syrup solids

confectioner's sugar

corn sweetener

corn syrup

corn syrup solids

crystalline fructose

date sugar

dextrin (a soluble carbohydrate from starch, used as an adhesive) dextrose (a liquid sugar solution—a form of glucose)

evaporated sugar cane

fructose (commonly found in honey and fruit—the sweetest of the simple sugars)

fruit juice concentrate

galactose (a white, crystalline, simple sugar dervied from milk sugar)

glucose (found in fruit and animal tissue—the basic sugar our bodies use; also called blood sugar)

granulated sugar

high-fructose corn syrup

honey

invert sugar

lactose (sugar derived from milk)

liquid cane sugar or syrup

maltose (a white, crystalline, water-soluble sugar derived from starch)

maple syrup

molasses

powdered sugar

raw sugar

sucrolose (molasses and glucose)

sucrose (white table sugar)

sugar cane syrup

table sugar

turbinado sugar

unrefined sugar

white sugar

Artificial Sweeteners

Americans consume 20 pounds of artificial sweeteners per person per year. Artificial sweeteners were originally designed for weight loss, but usage has proven that they increase appetite by stimulating the salivary glands, thus defeating their original purpose.[1]

Other research shows that none of these artificial

---

[1]S. D. Stellman and L. Garfinkel. "Artificial Sweetener Use and One Year Weight Change Among Women," *Preventive Medicine* 15 (March–April, 1986): 195–202.

sweeteners can be used without risk.[2] Here are brief summaries of sugar substitutes.

Saccharin (Sugar Twin, Sprinkle Twin, Sweet'n Low) is the original artificial sweetener and 300 times sweeter than sucrose (table sugar). It is used in baked goods, candy, canned fruit, chewing gum, dessert toppings, jams, soft drinks, medications and vitamins. Studies have linked saccharin with cancer in laboratory animals. Foods containing saccharin bear warning labels: "Use of this product may be hazardous to your health. This product contains saccharin, which has been determined to cause cancer in laboratory animals."

Aspartame (Equal, NutraSweet, NatraTaste) is 180 times sweeter than sucrose and is widely used in candy, cereal, frozen desserts, and soft drinks. Although some aspartame is used in commercial cooking, it is not wise to use it in home cooking because it is unstable at high temperatures.

Studies by Dr. Richard Wurtman of Massachusetts Institute of Technology have linked aspartame to many symptoms, including seizures, dizziness, visual impairment, disorientation, ear buzzing, a high level of SGOT (an enzyme that breaks down protein into amino acids) in the blood, tunnel vision, loss of equilibrium, sys-

[2]David Voreacos. "Experts Tell Panel of Continued Concern Over Use of Aspartame," *Los Angeles Times* (November 4, 1987): Part I, 9.

temic lupus, multiple sclerosis, headaches, fatigue, and Alzheimer's disease. A small group of people who have the rare hereditary disease phenylketonuria (PKU) must limit the use of aspartame, because they are unable to metabolize certain amino acids (phenylalaline—a by-product of aspartamene), which can result in mental retardation.

Acesulfame-K (Ace K, Sunnett, Sweet One) is 200 times sweeter than sucrose and is used in dry beverage mixes, candy, chewing gum, gelatins, and puddings. It is also combined with other sweeteners for use in fruit drinks and gelatin drinks. It is sometimes sold in packet or tablet form. Since acesulfame-K retains its sweetness when heated, it can be used for cooking and baking, unlike aspartame. It also has a slightly bitter aftertaste when used in large amounts. Tests show that this additive causes cancer in laboratory animals, which means it may increase cancer risk in humans.

Stevia is a small shrub in the chrysanthemum family, native to the highlands of South America. Stevia has a taste that is anywhere from 15 to 300 times sweeter than sucrose, depending on the way it is processed. It is available in the United States, mostly in health food stores, as a liquid concentrate or a powder. Some detect a licorice taste, and others find stevia leaves a slightly bitter aftertaste.

SucaFlore (combination of fructooligosacchride [FOS], soy extract, and potato starch) contains no sugar, but has a similar taste. A 3.4 gram serving has 3 grams of carbohydrates, and approximately 10 calories. SucaFlore is considered a dietary fiber. If eaten in large amounts, flatulence and some abdominal discomfort may occur. Studies in France show no long-term side effects with continued use.

Sucalose (Splenda) is 600 times sweeter than sucrose and is used in soda, chewing gum, baked goods, frozen desserts, non-alcoholic beverages, fruit juice, and gelatins. FDA pre-approval testing indicates potential toxicity. There have been no independent controlled studies and no long-term (12 to 24 months) human studies.

Sugar alcohol (Mannitol, Sorbitol, Xylitol, and Maltitol) is neither a "sugar" nor an "alcohol," and is not technically considered an artificial sweetener. These alcohols contain a little more than one-half of the carbohydrates in an equal amount of sugar and are produced commercially from carbohydrates, such as sucrose, glucose, and starch. They are used in ice cream, candy, cookies, chewing gum, and other sweet products in lieu of sugar. The government now requires labeling of these ingredients because they can cause side effects such as diarrhea and cramps.

Interesting Facts and Observations

Alcohol—While most alcohol has little or no sugar in its pure form (except cordials or after-dinner drinks), it takes the same pathway in the body that sugar does. Alcohol has such a simple chemistry that it passes directly into the bloodstream, much like a simple sugar.

Baby Food—After much thought, I decided not to include baby formulas and food in this book. When choosing food for infants, you must assess the nutritional value of individual brands in addition to the sugar content. A listing of this sort is beyond the scope of this book. Keep in mind, though, that sugar *is* added to many baby foods. (Beechnut is the only baby-food product that has no added sugar in any form.)

Calories—It is amazing how many calories creep into processed food, often because of added sugar and fat. There are typically 120 to 190 calories in 12 ounces of soda, virtually all from sugar! Start taking notice of calorie counts and don't waste your daily intake on sugar-laden junk foods. Vegetables have the least amount of calories and are full of vitamins and minerals. Try to include vegetables in each meal.

Carbohydrates—Sugar is the most concentrated form of carbohydrate. During digestion, carbohydrates are broken down into glucose and fructose. As glucose enters the bloodstream, the pancreas secretes insulin (a hormone), which in turn sends the glucose to cells for energy. When we eat too much sugar, the body cannot absorb all the glucose, and it is stored for later use or made into fat. The more sugar we eat, the harder the pancreas has to work, and, over time, the excess activity can lead to diabetes and other diseases.

Concentrated Fruit Juice—Concentrated fruit juice is used as a sweetener in many products—even those found in health food stores. Concentrated fruit juice has even more sugar than regular fruit juice. Stay away from it.

Forms of Sugar—Any word ending in "ose" (fructose, sucrose, glucose) is sugar, and there are many other words that basically translate to sugar. See "Sugar in All Its Forms" on page 15. When food, such as fruit and rice, is eaten in its natural form, the fiber in the food slows down digestion and metabolism, and the body is able to assimilate the sugar more easily.

Fried Foods—Many of the calories in processed foods come from either sugar or fat content. Fried foods are difficult to digest. The combination of sugar and fried fat in many products upsets the body chemistry with a one-two punch!

Fructose—Fructose is a simple sugar or monosaccharide. (Sucrose, or table sugar, is made up of 50 percent glucose and 50 percent fructose. Corn sweeteners contain about 80 percent fructose and 20 percent glucose.) It is found in fruits and all other carbohydrates in a natural form that the body can easily digest. Commonly sold at health food stores in white crystal form, fructose is used in most processed foods today and, therefore, largely contributes to the problem of daily excess sugar consumption. It increases the levels of cholesterol, lipoproteins (LDL), and very low lipoproteins (VLDP) in the body. Fructose depletes minerals, accelerates aging due to oxidative damage, and turns to fat far faster than glucose. Avoid processed fructose as much as possible.

Fruit Juices vs. Fresh Fruit—Unfortunately, fruit juice, whether it is freshly squeezed, frozen, or canned, without added sugar, has lots of simple sugar. Twelve ounces of freshly squeezed orange juice contains about same amount of sugar as a twelve-ounce soft drink. Research shows that freshly squeezed orange juice gets into the bloodstream just as fast, upsetting the body chemistry and suppressing the immune system. Grape juice and apple juice have almost as much sugar as orange juice. The best way to take advantage of the wonderful nutrient value of fruit is to eat it fresh and whole. This way you will get the fiber, and your body is able to process the sugar much more slowly.

Glycemic Index—Although it's not new, the glycemic index has recently become a very popular method for assessing carbohydrates. This rating system is based on a food's potential to raise blood sugar levels. The researchers who developed the index tested one carbohydrate at a time to see how quickly individuals were able to process the food, and how much blood sugar was raised when compared to an equal amount of pure glucose. The higher the glycemic index of a food, the faster the rise in blood sugar.

While the glycemic index is a useful tool to help make sense of carbohydrates, it can also cause confusion. For example, carrots and potatoes are relatively high on the glycemic index—higher in fact than some processed sugary foods such as ice cream and sugar-added cereals. This might lead you to believe that eating ice cream or frosted flakes is healthier than eating a carrot or a potato. However, there are other factors to consider. When you eat processed sugary foods, you upset your body chemistry, your body becomes acidic, some of the minerals become depleted and others become toxic, and the immune system becomes suppressed. Processed food is not healthier than carrots and potatoes. Carrots and potatoes eaten with protein and fat do not elevate blood glucose levels abnormally and make a healthy meal. The glycemic index may be a useful guide, but don't forget common sense!

Grams vs. Teaspoons—Most product labels list simple sugar content in grams—a unit of measure that means little to the average American. I find that the visual image of a teaspoon is much more helpful. Most people do not know how many grams are in one teaspoon of sugar so package labels are often meaningless. There are approximately four grams of sugar in one teaspoon. For example, most twelve-ounce soft drinks have approximately forty grams of sugar, the equivalent of ten teaspoons of sugar—ten teaspoons!

In this book, grams are rounded off to the nearest whole number, and teaspoons have been rounded off to quarter, half, and three-quarters of a teaspoon. For other measurement conversions, see page 28.

Homemade Recipes—When you make food at home from a recipe that calls for sugar, you might find it useful to convert the tablespoons or cups of sugar from the recipe into teaspoons from the measurement chart on page 28. Then you can divide the teaspoons by the number of servings you get out of the recipe to find out how many teaspoons are in an individual serving. You would be amazed by how much sugar is in homemade pies. Next time you make a sweet recipe, try cutting the sugar in half.

Food Labels—Every food product sold to the public in the United States must bear a label with the nutritional content of the product. The most plentiful ingredient is listed first, followed in sequential order to the last ingredient, which is found in the smallest amount. If there are three forms of sugar in a product, such as glucose, corn sweetener, and sucrose, the label can be deceiving. An example of this is jam. If the natural fruit content is listed first, followed by three forms of sugar, the jam probably contains more sugar than fruit, even though fruit is the first ingredient. The manufacturer lists the fruit first to make it look like the most plentiful ingredient, but in truth, the sugar collectively is the largest component of the product.

Hydrogenated Vegetable Oil—Many processed foods contain hydrogenated oils. Adding hydrogen to an oil changes it from a liquid to a solid, which adds texture to some food, but does nothing good for our bodies. Because the molecular structure of the oil is changed, it becomes more difficult to digest. Margarine is an example of hydrogenated oil. Studies have shown these fats and oils clog your arteries and can lead to heart problems.

Low-Fat and Nonfat (Fat-Free) Products—Many manufacturers have reduced the fat in their products, but to make them palatable, they have added sugar. Some common examples are potato chips, yogurt, cakes, muffins, coffee cake, and cookies. Carefully read product labels that say "less fat," "reduced fat," "nonfat," or "low fat." What manufacturers should be saying is "low fat, but high sugar!"

Natural Sugar vs. Added Sugar—When products have added sugar, it is impossible to tell what part of the total amount of sugar in the product comes from natural sugar versus that added from corn syrup, fructose, sucrose, glucose, or other forms of sugar.

Natural or Organic—Don't be fooled by the words "natural" or "organic" when it applies to sugar. Simple sugar is very concentrated sugar, whether it says natural, organic, or anything else.

Processed Foods—It's a good idea to stay away from processed foods as much as you can. Many are loaded with sugar, calories, chemicals, and fat, and have little fiber. Most are over-heated and processed, making them more difficult to digest, metabolize, and assimilate.

Sherbert, Sorbet, Ices, and Ice Cream—What's the difference between ice cream and sherbert, sorbet, and ices? Ice cream contains cream and/or milk. Sherbert usually contains milk and a form of fruit—usually fruit juice concentrate. Sorbet and ices contain fruit puree. Sherbert, sorbet, and ices have more sugar than ice cream—sometimes much more.

Table of Equivalent Measurements

4 grams of sugar = 1 teaspoon

Volume

1 tablespoon = 3 teaspoons

1 tablespoon = ½ fluid ounce

2 tablespoons = 1 fluid ounce

4 tablespoons = ¼ cup

¼ cup = 2 fluid ounces

⅓ cup = 5⅓ tablespoons

½ cup = 8 tablespoons

½ cup = 4 fluid ounces

⅔ cup = 10⅔ tablespoons

¾ cup = 6 fluid ounces

¾ cup = 12 tablespoons

1 cup = ½ pint

1 cup = 8 fluid ounces

1 cup = 16 tablespoons

1 pint = 2 cups

1 pint = 16 fluid ounces

1 quart = 2 pints

1 quart = 4 cups

1 quart = 32 fluid ounces

1 gallon = 4 quarts

1 gallon = 8 pints

Weight

½ ounce = 1 tablespoon

1 ounce = 28 grams

1 ounce = 2 tablespoons

2 ounces = ¼ cup

3.5 ounces = 100 grams

4 ounces = ½ cup

4 ounces = ¼ pound

4 ounces = 112 grams

8 ounces = ½ pound

8 ounces = 1 cup

8 ounces = 224 grams

12 ounces = ¾ pound

16 ounces = 1 pound

1 pound = 454 grams

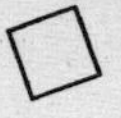

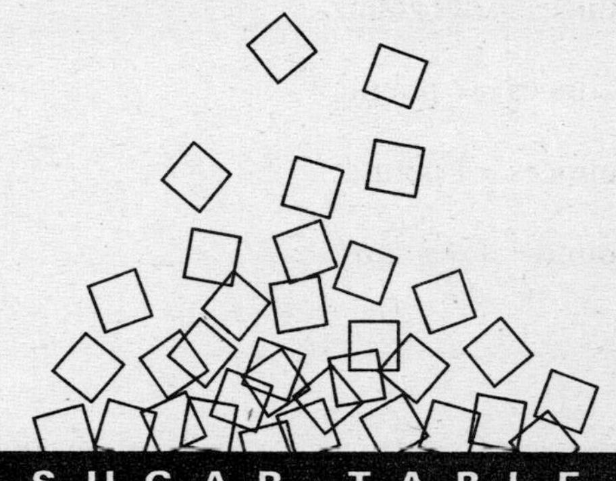

SUGAR TABLE

Although there may be sugar in many foods not mentioned in the sugar table, in general, foods with less than two teaspoons of sugar per serving are not included. Some examples are chewing gum, puffed cereals and corn flakes, bagels, and lemons. Since it would be virtually impossible to include all of the store brands from individual grocery chains, the most popular brand-name products are listed, which can be compared to the generic items you may purchase.

Within the body of the sugar table, the first column is labeled "Serving Size." Here, whenever possible, the most useful measurement (grams, ounces, fluid ounces, box size, pieces, single package serving, one cup, or one tablespoon) has been provided. This usually coincides with the manufacturer's example of one serving. Unfortunately, that portion size is often quite small and does not reflect the actual amount that you may consume at one time. When you start keeping track, you may notice that you eat double or triple the suggested serving size. So gauge your calories and sugar accordingly.

dbl = double

fl = fluid

g = gram

lb = pound

med = medium

oz = ounce

pkg = package

tbsp = tablespoon

tsps = teaspoons

w/ = with

w/o = without

FOOD	SERVING SIZE	CALORIES	CARBO-HYDRATES (GRAMS)	SUGAR (GRAMS)	SUGAR (TSPS)

BAKERY

Bars (Breakfast, Cereal, Diet, Energy, Fruit, Granola, Health, Nutrition, Power Snack, and Sport)

Most people think that granola bars are healthy products. While it is true that granola bars and other cereal bars contain many valuable nutrients, the sugar content (two to five teaspoons) interferes with their digestion by the body. Not only does the high sugar content make it more difficult to absorb the nutrients, but the nutrients can become toxic to the body. Unfortunately, many of these bars do not seem to be very healthy.

FOOD	SERVING SIZE	CALORIES	CARBO-HYDRATES (GRAMS)	SUGAR (GRAMS)	SUGAR (TSPS)
Boost					
Nutritional Energy Bar Chocolate Crunch	1.6 oz	190	29	16	4
Cap'n Crunch					
all varieties	0.8 oz	90	17	8	2
Carnation					
Chocolate Chip	1.3 oz	150	22	10	2½
Chocolate Chunk Granola	1.3 oz	389	61	28	7
Honey & Oats Granola	1.3 oz	130	23	9	2¼
Peanut Butter & Chocolate Chip	1.3 oz	150	21	10	2½
Health Valley					
Fat-Free Bakes, all varieties	1 bake	70	19	11	2¾
Fat-Free Breakfast Bakes, all varieties	1 bake	110	26	13	3¼
Fat-Free Fruit, all varieties	1 bar	140	35	14	3½
Fat-Free Granola, all varieties	1 bar	140	35	14	3½

FOOD	SERVING SIZE	CALORIES	CARBO-HYDRATES (GRAMS)	SUGAR (GRAMS)	SUGAR (TSPS)
Health Valley (continued)					
Fat-Free Marshmallow, all varieties	1 bar	100	24	11	2¾
Granola, Moist & Chewy, all varieties	1 bar	100–110	19–22	10–12	2½–3
Low-Fat Cereals, all varieties	1 bar	130	27–28	13–14	3¼–3½
Low-Fat Tarts, all varieties	1 bar	130	28	14	3½
Kellogg's					
Nutri-Grain Cereal Bars, all varieties	1.4 oz	140	27	13	3¼
Nutri-Grain Fruit Filled Squares, all varieties	1.7 oz	180–190	35	15–17	3¾–4¼
Nutri-Grain Twists, all varieties	1.4 oz	140	26–27	12–14	3–3½
Rice Krispies Treats Cereal Bars, all varieties	1 oz	90–110	16–18	7–9	1¾–2¼
Kudos					
Milk Chocolate w/ Snickers	1 bar	120	16	9	2¼
Chocolate Chip	1 bar	120	21	13	3¼
Peanut Butter	1 oz	130	19	13	3¼
Luna					
All flavors	1.7 oz	170–180	24–27	11–14	2¾–3½
Nature Valley					
All varieties	1.5 oz	180	29	11	2¾
Nature's Choice					
All varieties	1.3 oz	110–130	27–28	14	3½
Quaker					
All varieties	1 oz	110–120	20–23	9–11	2½–2¾
Slim Fast					
Dutch Chocolate	1.2 oz	140	20	13	3¼
Meal on the Go, all flavors	2 oz	220	35–36	20–23	5–5¾

FOOD	SERVING SIZE	CALORIES	CARBO-HYDRATES (GRAMS)	SUGAR (GRAMS)	SUGAR (TSPS)
Slim Fast (continued)					
Peanut Butter	1.2 oz	150	19	10	2½
Ultra Slim Fast Diet Bar Chewy Caramel	1 oz	120	22	11	2¾
Ultra Slim Fast Diet Bar Peanut Caramel Crunch	1 oz	120	22	18	4½
SnackWell's					
Banana Snack Bar	1.3 oz	130	27	16	4
Chewy Original	1 oz	110	22	14	3½
Fudge Dipped	1 oz	110	22	14	3½
Golden Snack Bar	1.3 oz	130	27	17	4¼
Strawberry Filling	1.3 oz	120	29	18	4½

Bread

Most plain bread has between one and two teaspoons of sugar per slice. Cinnamon bread and similar bread products contain more. Read labels.

Breakfast Rolls, Coffee Cakes, Danishes, Pastries, Tarts, Scones, and Turnovers

See also Cakes.

Mixes

FOOD	SERVING SIZE	CALORIES	CARBO-HYDRATES (GRAMS)	SUGAR (GRAMS)	SUGAR (TSPS)
Aunt Jemima					
Coffee Cake	⅓ cup (1.4 oz)	168	30	17	4¼
Betty Crocker					
Cinnamon Orange Bread	1/12 pkg	180	29	16	4
Cinnamon Streusel	¼ pkg	160	28	15	4¼
Pillsbury					
Chocoalte Chip Streusel	1/16 pkg	270	38	23	5¾

FOOD	SERVING SIZE	CALORIES	CARBO-HYDRATES (GRAMS)	SUGAR (GRAMS)	SUGAR (TSPS)
Ready to Eat					
Drake's					
Mini Coffee Cakes	4 cakes	220	33	20	5
Entenman's					
Banana Crunch coffee cake	2 oz	220	32	18	4½
Cinnamon Apple coffee cake, fat free	2 oz	130	29	16	4
Danish Light	⅛ cake	140	32	18	4½
French Crumb coffee cake	2 oz	210	29	15	4¾
Freihofer's					
Cinnamon Swirl Buns	1 (2.8 oz)	290	47	24	6
Coffee Cake Cinnamon Pecan	⅛ cake (2 oz)	220	33	20	5
Health Valley					
Fat-Free Healthy Scones, all varieties	1 scone	180	43	18	4½
Hostess					
Apple Tart	1 tart	400	47	22	5½
Coffee Cake Raspberry	1 cake	110	21	10	2½
Honey Bun Glazed	1 bun	320	35	21	5¼
Honey Bun Iced	1 bun	390	49	31	7¾
Kellogg's					
Eggo Toaster Muffins	2 oz	120–130	19–20	7–9	1¾–2¼
Pop-Tarts, plain, all varieties	1.8 oz	200–210	35–37	14–17	3½–4¼
Pop-Tarts Frosted, all varieties	1.8 oz	190–210	34–39	17–20	4¼–5
Pop-Tarts Snack-Stix, all varieties	2 oz	190	37	18	4½

FOOD	SERVING SIZE	CALORIES	CARBO-HYDRATES (GRAMS)	SUGAR (GRAMS)	SUGAR (TSPS)
Kellogg's (continued)					
Pop-Tarts Pastry Swirls, all varieties	2.5 oz	260	36–37	11–16	2¾–4
Pop-Tart Toaster Pastries, all varieties	2 oz	200–210	34–39	15–21	3¾–5¼
Little Debbie					
Coffee Cake Apple	1 pkg	220	36	22	5½
Coffee Cake Apple Streusel	1 pkg	220	37	23	5¾
Honey Bun	4 oz	510	53	23	5¾
Jelly Rolls	1 pkg	230	41	34	8¼
Nabisco					
Toastettes Tarts, all varieties	1.7 oz	190	35	17	4¼
Nature's Choice					
Toaster Pastries Low Fat, all varieties	1 pastry	180–200	36–42	16–24	4–6

Refrigerated or Frozen

FOOD	SERVING SIZE	CALORIES	CARBO-HYDRATES (GRAMS)	SUGAR (GRAMS)	SUGAR (TSPS)
Morton					
Honey Bun	1 bun	250	35	16	4
Honey Buns Mini	2 buns	360	38	12	3
Pepperidge Farms					
Apple Turnover	3 oz	330	48	35	8¾
Apple Turnover, mini	1.4 oz	140	15	10	2½
Apple w/ Vanilla Icing Turnover	3.4 oz	380	53	37	9¼
Blueberry Turnover	3.1 oz	340	45	35	8¾
Cherry Turnover	3.1 oz	320	46	36	8
Peach Turnover	3.1 oz	340	47	31	7¾
Raspberry Turnover	3.1 oz	330	47	33	8¼

FOOD	SERVING SIZE	CALORIES	CARBO-HYDRATES (GRAMS)	SUGAR (GRAMS)	SUGAR (TSPS)
Pillsbury					
Sweet Roll, all varieties	1 roll	140–170	23–26	9–11	2¼–2¾
Grands Sweet Roll, all varieties	1 roll	300–340	52–54	22–24	5½–6
Turnovers, all varieties	1 turnover	170	23	11–12	3¾–4

Brownies and Fudge

Mixes

FOOD	SERVING SIZE	CALORIES	CARBO-HYDRATES (GRAMS)	SUGAR (GRAMS)	SUGAR (TSPS)
Arrowhead Mills					
Brownie Mix, all varieties	1 brownie	110–120	26–28	20–22	5–5½
Betty Crocker					
Brownie w/ Mini Kisses	⅙ pkg	220	36	27	6¾
Dark Chocolate Brownie	⅑ pkg	190	27	19	4¾
Frosted, all varieties	1/20 pkg	210	30–31	22–23	5½–5¾
Fudge Brownie	⅑ pkg	190	27	19	4¾
All other varieties of brownie and fudge	1/20 pkg	170–210	23–29	15–21	3¾–5¼
Betty Crocker Sweet Rewards					
Brownie Mix, low fat	1/18 pkg	130	27	18	4½
Brownie Mix, reduced fat	1/20 pkg	150	27	19	4¾
Duncan Hines					
Chewy Fudge Brownie Mix (snack size)	½ pkg	120	24	16	4
Chewy Fudge Premium Brownie (family size)	1/20 pkg	120	25	17	4¼
Dark 'N Fudgy Chocolate Lover's Premium Brownie	1/18 pkg	120	25	18	4½
Double Fudge Chocolate Lover's Premium Brownie	1/20 pkg	140	28	19	4¾
Milk Chocolate Chunk Brownie Mix	1/20 pkg	140	26	20	5

FOOD	SERVING SIZE	CALORIES	CARBO-HYDRATES (GRAMS)	SUGAR (GRAMS)	SUGAR (TSPS)
Duncan Hines (continued)					
Mississippi Mud Chocolate Lover's Premium Brownie	1/20 pkg	130	27	19	4¾
Raspberry Fudge Chocolate Lover's Premium Brownie	1/20 pkg	120	23	16	4
Pillsbury					
Brownie Mix, Fudge (15 oz box)	1/16 pkg	110	22	15	3¾
Brownie Mix, Fudge (19.5 oz box)	1/18 pkg	130	26	18	4½
Thick 'n Fudgy Cheesecake Swirl	1/18 pkg	110	19	13	3¼
Thick 'n Fudgy Chocolate Chunk	1/16 pkg	120	22	15	3¾
Thick 'n Fudgy Double Chocolate	1/16 pkg	120	23	15	3¾
Thick 'n Fudgy Caramel Swirl	1/14 pkg	120	23	15	3¾
Thick 'n Fudgy Hot Fudge Swirl	1/14 pkg	130	23	16	4
Thick 'n Fudgy Walnut	1/12 pkg	140	24	15	3¾
Robin Hood					
Gold Medal Pouch Fudge	1/10 pkg	170	24	17	4¼
Weight Watchers					
Brownie a la Mode	1 brownie	190	33	15	3¾
Double Fudge Parfait Brownie	2.7 oz	95	20	9	2¼

Ready to Eat

FOOD	SERVING SIZE	CALORIES	CARBO-HYDRATES (GRAMS)	SUGAR (GRAMS)	SUGAR (TSPS)
Betty Crocker Sweet Rewards					
Brownie Snack Bar, fat free	1.1 oz	100	24	16	4
Double Fudge Supreme Snack Bar, fat free	1.1 oz	100	25	15	3¾

FOOD	SERVING SIZE	CALORIES	CARBO-HYDRATES (GRAMS)	SUGAR (GRAMS)	SUGAR (TSPS)
Entenmann's					
Brownies Little Bites Fudge	3 pieces	290	37	26	6½
Little Debbie					
Brownie Light	1.9 oz	185	39	27	6¼
Fudge	2.2 oz	269	39	24	6
Pillsbury					
Fudge Brownie	1⁄12 pkg	180	25	16	4

Cakes

When calculating the grams of sugar in a piece of cake that you have prepared from a mix, do not forget to include the sugar content of the frosting. See Dessert Frostings and Toppings on page 157.

Mixes

FOOD	SERVING SIZE	CALORIES	CARBO-HYDRATES (GRAMS)	SUGAR (GRAMS)	SUGAR (TSPS)
Betty Crocker					
Gingerbread Cake & Cookie Mix	⅛ pkg	230	39	18	4½
Pineapple Upside Down Cake	⅙ pkg	400	64	43	10¾
Pound Cake	⅛ pkg	260	45	26	6½
Betty Crocker Sweet Rewards					
Fat Free Snack	⅛ pkg	160–170	38–39	21–27	5¼–6¾
Reduced Fat, all varieties	1⁄12 pkg	200–210	35–36	20–21	5–5¼
Duncan Hines					
Moist Deluxe					
Angel	1⁄12 pkg	140	31	23	5¾
Banana Supreme	1⁄12 pkg	180	36	22	5½
Butter Recipe Fudge Supreme	1⁄10 pkg	220	40	28	7
Butter Recipe Golden Supreme	1⁄12 pkg	230	42	29	7¼

FOOD	SERVING SIZE	CALORIES	CARBO-HYDRATES (GRAMS)	SUGAR (GRAMS)	SUGAR (TSPS)
Moist Deluxe (continued)					
Butterscotch Premium	1/12 pkg	180	36	22	5½
Caramel	1/12 pkg	180	36	22	5½
Chocolate Mocha Premium	1/12 pkg	180	34	20	5
Dark Chocolate Fudge	1/12 pkg	180	34	20	5
Devil's Food	1/12 pkg	180	34	20	5
French Vanilla	1/12 pkg	180	36	22	5½
Fudge Marble	1/12 pkg	180	36	22	5½
Lemon Supreme	1/12 pkg	180	36	22	5½
Orange Supreme	1/12 pkg	180	36	22	5½
Pineapple Supreme	1/12 pkg	180	36	22	5½
Strawberry Supreme	1/12 pkg	180	36	22	5½
Swiss Chocolate	1/12 pkg	180	34	20	5
White	1/12 pkg	170	34	20	5
Wild Cherry Vanilla Premium	1/12 pkg	180	36	22	5½
Yellow	1/12 pkg	180	36	22	5½
General Mills					
Stir & Bake, all varieties	1/6 pkg	240–250	42–47	26–30	6½–7½
SuperMoist					
Angel Food, all varieties	1/12 pkg	140	32	24	6
Butter Chocolate	1/12 pkg	125	35	21	5¼
Butter Pecan	1/12 pkg	240	35	20	5
Butter Yellow	1/12 pkg	260	36	20	5
Carrot Cake	1/10 pkg	320	42	25	6¼
Cherry Chip	1/10 pkg	300	41	23	5¾
Chocolate Chip	1/12 pkg	250	35	20	5
Chocolate Fudge	1/12 pkg	270	35	21	5¼

FOOD	SERVING SIZE	CALORIES	CARBO-HYDRATES (GRAMS)	SUGAR (GRAMS)	SUGAR (TSPS)
SuperMoist (continued)					
Chocolate w/Creamy Swirls of Fudge	1/9 pkg	210	32	18	4½
Devils Food	1/12 pkg	270	35	21	5¼
Double Chocolate Swirl	1/12 pkg	270	35	21	5¼
Easy Angel Food	¼ pkg	170	37	23	5¾
French Vanilla	1/12 pkg	240	35	20	5
Fudge Marble	1/10 pkg	290	43	25	6¼
German Chocolate	1/12 pkg	270	36	21	5¼
Golden Vanilla	1/12 pkg	240	35	20	5
Lemon	1/12 pkg	240	36	20	5
Milk Chocolate	1/12 pkg	240	34	20	5
Party Swirl	1/12 pkg	250	35	19	4¾
Pineapple	1/12 pkg	250	35	20	5
Rainbow Chip	1/10 pkg	300	41	23	5¾
Sour Cream White	1/10 pkg	280	41	22	5½
Spice	1/12 pkg	240	35	20	5
Strawberry	1/12 pkg	250	35	21	5¼
Strawberry Swirl	1/10 pkg	300	41	23	5¾
White	1/12 pkg	230	34	18	4½
White Chocolate Swirl	1/12 pkg	250	34	19	4¾
Yellow	1/12 pkg	250	25	20	5
Yellow w/Creamy Swirls of Fudge	1/9 pkg	210	32	18	4½
Pillsbury					
Angel Food	1/12 pkg	140	31	23	5¾
Gingerbread	1/8 pkg	220	40	20	5
Moist Supreme, all varieties	1/12 pkg	240–270	33–36	17–21	4¼–5¼

FOOD	SERVING SIZE	CALORIES	CARBO-HYDRATES (GRAMS)	SUGAR (GRAMS)	SUGAR (TSPS)
Ready to Eat					
Baby Watson					
Cheesecake	1/16 cake	390	23	20	5
Cheesecake Light	1/16 cake	280	24	18	4½
Creole Royal Pineapple Apricot	1/16 cake	290	20	15	3¾
Carousel New York Cheesecake	1/16 cake	250	16	15	3¾
Entenmann's					
Banana Crunch	1.9 oz	140	33	20	5
Banana Loaf	2 oz	150	23	14	3½
Blueberry Crunch	2 oz	140	32	18	4½
Butter	2 oz	220	31	18	4½
Carrot Cake	2.5 oz	290	35	26	6½
Chocolate Chip	2 oz	130	31	19	4¾
Chocolate Crunch	1.8 oz	130	20	10	2½
Chocolate Fudge Iced	3 oz	210	51	39	9¾
Chocolate Loaf	1.9 oz	130	30	18	4½
Mocha Iced	3 oz	200	46	32	8
Marble	1.8 oz	130	29	18	4½
Raisin	2 oz	220	32	21	5¼
Spice Apple	1.9 oz	130	30	19	4¾
Freihofer's					
Angel Food	1/5 cake	150	35	23	5¾
Crumb	1/8 cake	240	33	13	3¼
Homestyle Golden Loaf Pound	1/8 cake	200	28	17	4¼
Pound	1/5 cake	330	41	24	6

FOOD	SERVING SIZE	CALORIES	CARBO-HYDRATES (GRAMS)	SUGAR (GRAMS)	SUGAR (TSPS)
Greenfield Blondie					
Apple Spice	1 piece	120	28	20	5
Chocolate Chip	1 piece	120	29	21	5¼
Hostess					
Angel Food Ring	⅙ cake	150	29	19	4¾
Apple Twist	1 twist	220	42	16	4
Baseball Yellow Cakes	1 cake	160	32	19	4¾
Choco Licious	1 cake	170	28	17	4¼
Choco-Diles	1 cake	240	33	22	5½
Crumb Cake	1 cake	210	33	16	4
Cup Cakes Chocolate	1 cake	180	30	17	4¼
Cup Cakes Chocolate Light	1 cake	140	29	19	4¾
Cup Cakes Orange	1 cake	160	27	20	5
Dessert Cups	1 cup	90	18	8	2
Ding Dongs	2 cakes	370	46	33	8¼
Fruit Cake Holiday	⅙ cake	490	93	39	9¾
Fruit Loaf	1 loaf	350	67	28	7
Ho Ho's	2 cakes	250	34	23	5¾
Holiday Cakes	1 cake	160	31	19	4¾
Hopper Cakes	1 cake	160	32	19	4¾
Lights Low Fat Cinnamon Crumb Cake	1 cake	90	19	16	4
Lil Angels	1 cake	90	17	11	2¾
Pecan Spinners	1 cake	110	15	8	2
Pound Cake	⅕ cake	350	48	22	5½
Snow Balls	1 cake	160	29	17	4¼
Suzy Q's	1 cake	220	35	21	5¼
Suzy Q's Banana	1 cake	220	32	18	4½

FOOD	SERVING SIZE	CALORIES	CARBO-HYDRATES (GRAMS)	SUGAR (GRAMS)	SUGAR (TSPS)
Hostess (continued)					
Swirls Caramel Pecan	1 cake	140	25	10	2½
Tiger Tails	1 cake	160	26	14	3½
Twinkies	1 cake	150	25	14	3½
Twinkies Banana	2 cakes	300	42	24	6
Twinkies Devil Food	2 cakes	300	47	28	7
Twinkies Light	1 cake	120	24	15	3¾
Twinkies Strawberry Fruit 'n Creme	1 piece	150	30	17	4¼
Jell-O					
Cheesecake Snack Original	1 snack	160	23	19	4¾
Cheesecake Snack Strawberry	1 snack	150	26	23	5¾
Little Debbie					
Apple Flips	1 pkg	150	24	13	3¼
Chocolate Marshmallow Pie	1 pie	160	27	16	4
Coconut Rounds	1 pkg	140	22	14	3½
Devil Cremes	1.6 oz	190	28	20	5
Devil Squares	1 pkg	260	31	29	7¼
Easter Basket Cakes	1 pkg	310	44	35	8¾
Fancy Cakes	1 pkg	300	44	34	8½
Fudge Crispy	1 pkg	170	20	13	3¼
Fudge Rounds	1.2 oz	140	23	14	3½
Golden Cremes	1.5 oz	170	25	18	4½
Holiday Cake Vanilla	1 pkg	210	44	35	8¾
Marshmallow Crispy Bars	1 bar	140	26	13	3¼
Nutly Bar	2 bars	310	32	20	5
Oatmeal Creme Pie	1 pie	170	26	14	3½
Pecan Twins Spin Wheels	1 pkg	110	16	7	1¾

FOOD	SERVING SIZE	CALORIES	CARBO-HYDRATES (GRAMS)	SUGAR (GRAMS)	SUGAR (TSPS)
Little Debbie (continued)					
Pumpkin Delights	1 pkg	130	21	12	3
Smiley Faces Cherry	1 pkg	140	23	13	3¼
Snack Cake Chocolate	1 pkg	300	23	33	8¼
Snack Cake Vanilla	1 pkg	320	45	36	9
Spice	1 pkg	300	43	35	8¾
Star Crunch	1 pkg	140	21	15	3¾
Swiss Rolls	2 cakes	270	38	25	6¼
Teddy Berries	1 pkg	130	23	12	3
Vanilla	1 pkg	370	53	42	10½
Vanilla Cremes	1 pkg	170	25	18	4½
Zebra Cakes	1 pkg	150	45	36	9
Nabisco					
Frosted Strawberry	1 cake	190	36	17	4¼
Nature's Choice					
Fat Free, all varieties	1 cake	180	41	21	5¼
Pepperidge Farm					
Coconut Layer	2.9 oz	300	41	22	5½
Lemon Mousse	2.5 oz	250	34	21	5¼
Strawberry Cream w/Coconut	2.7 oz	230	38	23	5¾
Vaniila	2.9 oz	290	41	23	5¾
Yellow layer	2.9 oz	290	40	36	9
Penguin					
Pannettone Au Beurre	⅙ cake	310	47	21	5¼
Sara Lee					
Banana	⅙ cake	230	37	28	7
Banana Sundae	⅒ cake	270	32	24	6
Carrot	⅙ cake	320	39	35	8¾

FOOD	SERVING SIZE	CALORIES	CARBO-HYDRATES (GRAMS)	SUGAR (GRAMS)	SUGAR (TSPS)
Sara Lee (continued)					
Cheesecake Cherry	¼ cake	350	55	35	8¾
Cheesecake Chocolate Chip	¼ cake	410	47	43	10¾
Cheesecake Chocolate Mousse	⅕ cake	400	37	27	6¾
Cheesecake French	⅙ cake	350	34	22	5½
Cheesecake Singles Fudge Brownie Crumble	1 slice	400	43	36	9
Cheesecake Singles Strawberry Drizzle	1 slice	380	46	40	10
Cheesecake Strawberry	¼ cake	330	49	36	9
Cheesecake Strawberry French	⅙ cake	320	43	26	6½
Cheesecake Bars Chocolate Dipped Original	1 bar	190	14	12	3
Cheesecake Bites Chocolate Praline Pecan	5 bites	480	44	33	8¼
Cheesecake Bites Toasted Almond Crunch	5 bites	470	43	24	6
Harvest Pumpkin Spice	⅛ cake	270	33	25	6¼
Layer Cake Coconut	⅛ cake	280	34	25	6¼
Layer Cake Double Chocolate	⅛ cake	260	33	28	7
Layer Cake Fudge Golden	⅛ cake	270	36	30	7½
Layer Cake German Chocolate	⅛ cake	280	36	30	7½
Layer Cake Vanilla	⅛ cake	250	31	25	6¼
Original Cheesecake Reduced Fat	¼ cake	310	40	28	7
Pound Cake	¼ cake	320	38	21	5¼

FOOD	SERVING SIZE	CALORIES	CARBO-HYDRATES (GRAMS)	SUGAR (GRAMS)	SUGAR (TSPS)
Sara Lee (continued)					
Pound Cake Chocolate Swirl	¼ cake	110	14	11	2¾
Pound Cake Family Size	⅙ cake	310	36	15	3¾
Pound Cake Free & Light	¼ cake	200	39	21	5¼
Pound Cake Golden	¼ cake	120	15	11	2¾
Pound Cake Reduced Fat	¼ cake	100	15	10	2½
Pound Cake Strawberry	¼ cake	290	44	25	6¼
Red White & Blueberry	⅒ cake	210	31	21	5¼
Strawberry Shortcake	⅛ cake	180	27	15	3¾
Tastykake					
Butter Cream, mini	2 pieces (1 oz)	110	18	12	3
Butterscotch Iced	1 oz	183	20	12	3
Chocolate Cup Cake	1 oz	110	20	12	3
Chocolate, mini	2 pieces (1 oz)	110	18	12	3
Chocolate	2 pieces (1.4 oz)	180	24	18	4½
Chocolate Cream Cup Cake	1.2 oz	125	21	13	3¼
Chocolate Cream Filled Iced	1.8 oz	188	30	17	4¼
Chocolate Creamies	1.5 oz	180	26	17	4¼
Coconut	1.7 oz	87	11	8	2
Creme Filled, mini	2 pieces (1 oz)	110	16	10	2½
Jelly Filled	1 oz	93	19	11	2¾
Kreme Kup	0.9 oz	95	16	10	2½
Peanut Butter	0.7 oz	90	11	8	2
Sprinkled Creamies	1.4 oz	150	25	14	3½

FOOD	SERVING SIZE	CALORIES	CARBO-HYDRATES (GRAMS)	SUGAR (GRAMS)	SUGAR (TSPS)
Tastykake (continued)					
Vanilla Cream Filled	1.2 oz	105	21	10	2½
Vanilla Creamies	1.5 oz	190	26	18	4½
Whitchy Good Treat	.25 oz	150	24	14	3½
Weight Watchers					
Almond Amaretto Cheesecake	3 oz	170	23	12	3
Brownie Cheesecake	3.5 oz	200	32	11	2¾
Double Fudge	2.7 oz	190	36	22	5½
Triple Chocolate	3.1 oz	199	32	20	5

Cookies

There are so many different types of cookies on the market. You'll find that many manufacturers list the nutritional facts for just one cookie on the label. But who can eat just one cookie? Keep track of how many cookies you eat (and the teaspoons of sugar you are consuming), and chances are you'll be amazed.

Dough, Refrigerated or Frozen

FOOD	SERVING SIZE	CALORIES	CARBO-HYDRATES (GRAMS)	SUGAR (GRAMS)	SUGAR (TSPS)
Mrs. Field's					
Semi Sweet Chocolate Chip	1/12 pkg	161	21	10	2½
Semi Sweet Chocolate Chip Walnut	1/12 pkg	270	32	23	5¾
Nestlé					
Toll House Chocolate Chip	2 tbsp	60	20	12	3
Chocolate Chip w/ Fudge	2 tbsp	150	21	12	3
Toll House Walnut Chocolate Chip & Peanut Butter	1/20 pkg	110	14	8	2
Toll House Sugar Cookies	1/20 pkg	110	15	8	2

FOOD	SERVING SIZE	CALORIES	CARBO-HYDRATES (GRAMS)	SUGAR (GRAMS)	SUGAR (TSPS)
Pillsbury					
Dough Mix, all flavors (18-oz box)	1 oz	120–140	16–19	9–11	2¼–2¾
Dough Mix, reduced fat, all flavors	1 oz	110	19	12	4

Mixes

FOOD	SERVING SIZE	CALORIES	CARBO-HYDRATES (GRAMS)	SUGAR (GRAMS)	SUGAR (TSPS)
Arrowhead Mills					
Chocolate Chip, regular and wheat-free	1 cookie	80	16	9	2¼
Oatmeal Raisin	1 cookie	80	16	9	2¼
Betty Crocker					
Chocolate, all varieties	3 tbsp	150–160	20–21	12–14	3–3½
Chocolate Peanut Butter Bars	1/12 pkg	200	26	18	4½
Date Bars	1/12 pkg	150	18	14	3½
Easy Layer Dessert Bars	1/16 pkg	140	21	12	3
Hershey Cookie Bars	1/16 pkg	150	21	14	3½
Peanut Butter	3 tbsp	160	20	12	3
Sugar	3 tbsp	160	22	13	2¼
Sunkist Lemon Bars	1/16 pkg	140	24	17	4¼
Supreme Dessert Bar Mix	1/16 pkg	164	23	14	3½
Duncan Hines					
Chocolate Chip	1/24 pkg	140	22	14	3½
Golden Sugar	1/24 pkg	110	21	12	3
Peanut Butter	1/24 pkg	120	16	9	2¼
Estee					
Chocolate Chip	3 cookies	130	17	10	2½
Nestlé					
Oatmeal Scotchies	2 tbsp	50	20	11	2¾
Peanut Butter Chocolate Chip	2 tbsp	70	19	12	3

FOOD	SERVING SIZE	CALORIES	CARBO-HYDRATES (GRAMS)	SUGAR (GRAMS)	SUGAR (TSPS)
Pillsbury					
Cookie Mix, all varieties	3 tbsp	140–150	21	12–13	3–3¼

Ready to Eat

FOOD	SERVING SIZE	CALORIES	CARBO-HYDRATES (GRAMS)	SUGAR (GRAMS)	SUGAR (TSPS)
Archway					
Almond Crescent	4 cookies	200	34	12	3
Apple n' Raisin	1 cookie	130	20	11	2¾
Apricot Filled	1 cookie	110	18	9	2½
Bells & Stars	6 cookies	300	38	14	3½
Blueberry Filled	1 cookie	110	19	14	3½
Carrot Cake	1 cookie	120	18	14	3½
Cherry Filled	1 cookie	110	19	14	3½
Cherry Nougat	3 cookies	150	18	12	3
Chocolate Chip	2 cookies	260	38	18	4½
Chocolate Chip & Toffee	2 cookies	280	36	18	4½
Chocolate Chip Bag	3 cookies	130	17	9	2¼
Chocolate Chip Drop	1 cookie	140	11	9	2¼
Chocolate Chip Ice Box	1 cookie	140	19	9	2¼
Chocolate Chip Mini	12 cookies	150	20	9	2¼
Cinnamon Snaps	12 cookies	150	19	9	2¼
Coconut Macaroon	1 cookie	90	14	9	2¼
Cookie Jar Hermits	1 cookie	110	19	9	2¼
Dark Chocolate	2 cookies	220	40	14	3½
Dutch Chocolate	1 cookie	120	19	13	3¼
Fig Bar, low fat	2 cookies	100	23	12	3
Frosty Lemon	1 cookie	120	19	15	3¾
Frosty Orange	1 cookie	120	19	8	2
Fruit & Honey Bar	1 cookie	110	18	14	3½

FOOD	SERVING SIZE	CALORIES	CARBO-HYDRATES (GRAMS)	SUGAR (GRAMS)	SUGAR (TSPS)
Archway (continued)					
Fruit Bar, fat free	1 cookie	90	21	11	2¾
Fruit Cake	1 cookie	140	20	12	3
Fudge Nut, Bar	1 cookie	120	17	8	2
Fun Chip Mini	12 cookies	140	21	9	2¼
Gingersnaps	5 cookies	130	22	12	3
Granola No Fat	2 cookies	100	22	14	3½
Holiday Pak	2 cookies	150	19	9	2¼
Ice Box	2 cookies	280	36	18	4½
Iced Gingerbread	3 cookies	149	23	10	2½
Iced Molasses	1 cookie	110	19	8	2
Iced Oatmeal	1 cookie	120	19	15	3¾
Lemon Snaps	12 cookies	150	19	9	2¼
Malted Nougat	3 cookies	160	17	11	2¾
New Orleans Cake	1 cookie	110	18	8	2
Nutty Nougat	6 cookies	320	36	14	3½
Oatmeal	2 cookies	220	38	20	5
Oatmeal Apple Filled	1 cookie	110	18	14	2½
Oatmeal Date Filled	1 cookie	110	18	15	3¾
Oatmeal Mini	24 cookies	300	38	14	3½
Oatmeal Pecan	2 cookies	240	36	18	4½
Oatmeal Raisin	2 cookies	220	38	26	6½
Oatmeal Raisin Bran	2 cookies	220	38	18	4½
Old Fashioned Molasses	2 cookies	240	40	20	5
Old Fashioned Windmill	2 cookies	200	30	18	4½
Party Treats	3 cookies	140	20	9	2¼
Peanut Butter	2 cookies	280	32	16	4

FOOD	SERVING SIZE	CALORIES	CARBO-HYDRATES (GRAMS)	SUGAR (GRAMS)	SUGAR (TSPS)
Archway (continued)					
Peanut Butter & Chip	3 cookies	130	16	8	2
Peanut Butter Nougat	3 cookies	160	18	8	2
Pecan Crunch	6 cookies	150	18	8	2
Pfeffermusse	2 cookies	140	32	22	5½
Pineapple Filled	1 cookie	100	16	8	2
Raisin Oatmeal	1 cookie	130	19	9	2¼
Raisin Oatmeal Bag	3 cookies	130	19	9	2¼
Raspberry Filled	1 cookie	110	18	9	2¼
Rocky Road	1 cookie	130	18	9	2¼
Ruth Golden Oatmeal	1 cookie	120	19	11	2¾
Select Assortment	3 cookies	130	18	9	2¼
Soft Molasses Drop	2 cookies	220	36	12	3
Soft Sugar	2 cookies	220	26	22	5½
Strawberry Filled	1 cookie	110	18	9	2¼
Sugar	2 cookies	240	40	22	5½
Vanilla Wafers	5 cookies	130	22	15	3¾
Wedding Cakes	3 cookies	160	20	9	2¼
Bakery Wagon					
Apple Walnut Raisin	2 cookies	200	32	16	4
Cobbler Apple Cranberry, fat free	2 cookies	140	32	20	5
Cobbler Apple, fat free	2 cookies	140	34	18	4½
Cobbler Mixed Fruit, fat free	2 cookies	140	32	22	5½
Cobbler Raspberry, fat free	2 cookies	140	34	14	3½
Ginger Snaps	5 cookies	160	22	10	2½

FOOD	SERVING SIZE	CALORIES	CARBO-HYDRATES (GRAMS)	SUGAR (GRAMS)	SUGAR (TSPS)
Bakery Wagon (continued)					
Honey Fruit Bars	1 cookie	100	17	8	2
Iced Molasses	1 cookie	100	18	9	2¼
Iced Molasses Mini	3 cookies	130	18	12	3
Oatmeal Apple Filled	2 cookies	180	28	14	2½
Oatmeal Chocolate Chunk	2 cookies	200	32	8	2
Oatmeal Date Filled	2 cookies	180	34	10	2½
Oatmeal Raspberry Filled	2 cookies	200	32	14	3½
Oatmeal Soft	2 cookies	200	32	20	5
Oatmeal Walnut Raisin	2 cookies	200	34	8	2
Vanilla Wafers, cholesterol free	2 cookies	260	44	28	7
Barbara					
Animal Cookies Vanilla	16 cookies	260	40	8	2
Chocolate Chip	2 cookies	160	20	10	2½
Double Dutch Chocolate	2 cookies	160	20	10	2½
Fig Bars, fat free, all flavors	1 cookie	60	15	11	2¾
Fig Bars, low fat, all flavors	1 cookie	60	14	9	2¼
Homestyle Chewy Chocolate, fat free	2 cookies	80	20	11	2¾
Homestyle Chocolate Mint, fat free	2 cookies	80	20	12	3
Homestyle Nutt'n Crispies, fat free	2 cookies	80	20	11	2¾
Homestyle Oatmeal Raisin, fat free	2 cookies	80	20	12	3
Mini Caramel Apple, fat free	6 cookies	110	24	12	3
Mini Cocoa Mocha, fat free	6 cookies	100	23	11	2¾

FOOD	SERVING SIZE	CALORIES	CARBO-HYDRATES (GRAMS)	SUGAR (GRAMS)	SUGAR (TSPS)
Barbara (continued)					
Mini Double Chocolate, fat free	6 cookies	100	23	12	3
Mini Oatmeal Raisin	6 cookies	110	24	12	3
Old Fashioned Oatmeal	2 cookies	140	22	10	2½
Snackimals, all flavors	8 cookies	120	18	8	2
Traditional Shortbread	3 cookies	240	30	9	2¼
Barnum's					
Animal Crackers	12 cookies	140	23	8	2
Animal Crackers Chocolate	10 cookies	130	23	8	2
Betty Crocker Sweet Rewards					
Fat-Free Snack Bars, all varieties	1 cookie	120	24–29	15–19	3¾–4¾
Biscos					
Sugar Wafers	8 cookies	140	21	13	3¼
Waffle Cremes	4 cookies	180	24	17	4¼
Chip-Ahoy					
Bite-size Chocolate Chip	14 cookies	170	21	10	2½
Chewy Chocolate Chip	3 cookies	170	23	14	3½
Chunky Chocolate Chip	2 cookies	160	22	14	3½
Real Chocolate Chip, reduced fat	3 cookies	160	21	10	2½
Sprinkled Real Chocolate Chip	3 cookies	170	24	12	3
Striped Chocolate Chip	2 cookies	160	20	12	3
Chortles					
Cookies, all varieties	½ pkg	125	23	11	2¾
Cookie Lover's					
Blue Ribbon Brownies	2 cookies	180	28	14	3½
Classic Shortbread	2 cookies	220	24	8	2
Dutch Chocolate Chip	2 cookies	180	24	8	2

FOOD	SERVING SIZE	CALORIES	CARBO-HYDRATES (GRAMS)	SUGAR (GRAMS)	SUGAR (TSPS)
Cookie Lover's (continued)					
Fancy Peanut Butter	2 cookies	100	20	8	2
Grahams Cinnamon Honey	4 cookies	220	48	12	3
Grahams Honey	4 cookies	200	44	10	2½
One-Time Raisin	2 cookies	180	28	12	3
Delacres					
Assortment	4 cookies	130	18	10	2½
Dutch Mill					
Chocolate Chip	3 cookies	160	18	10	2½
Coconut Macaroons	3 cookies	120	14	12	3
Oatmeal Raisin	3 cookies	130	18	10	2½
Estee					
Chocolate Chip	8 cookies	300	42	10	2½
Coconut	8 cookies	280	38	10	2½
Creme Wafers Chocolate	7 cookies	160	21	9	2¼
Creme Wafers Lemon	5 cookies	170	23	10	2½
Creme Wafers Peanut Butter	5 cookies	170	21	7	1¾
Creme Wafers Triple Decker Banana Split	3 cookies	140	18	8	2
Creme Wafers Triple Decker Chocolate, Caramel & Peanut Butter	3 cookies	140	17	7	1¾
Creme Wafer Vanilla	7 cookies	160	22	7	1¾
Creme Wafer Vanilla & Strawberry	5 cookies	170	23	10	2½
Fig Bars Apple, low fat	2 cookies	100	22	14	3½
Fig Bars Cranberry, low fat	2 cookies	100	22	14	3½
Fig Bars, low fat	2 cookies	100	23	13	3¼
Fudge	8 cookies	300	38	10	2½

FOOD	SERVING SIZE	CALORIES	CARBO-HYDRATES (GRAMS)	SUGAR (GRAMS)	SUGAR (TSPS)
Estee (continued)					
Lemon	8 cookies	280	38	10	2½
Oatmeal Raisin	8 cookies	260	38	12	3
Sandwich Chocolate	3 cookies	160	24	9	2¼
Sandwich Original	3 cookies	160	24	10	2½
Sandwich Vanilla	6 cookies	320	50	14	3½
Shortbread, reduced fat	8 cookies	260	44	10	2½
Vanilla	8 cookies	280	38	10	2½
Famous Amos					
Chocolate & Pecan	4 cookies	140	17	9	2¼
Chocolate Chip	4 cookies	130	18	10	2½
Freihofer's					
Chocolate Chip	4 cookies	240	36	20	5
Girl Scout					
Animal Treasures	2 cookies	190	25	12	3
Caramel deLites	2 cookies	140	19	13	3¼
Lemon Pastry Cremes	3 cookies	130	22	13	3¼
Peanut Butter Patties	2 cookies	150	16	9	2¼
Peanut Butter Sandwiches	3 cookies	180	23	14	3½
Short Bread	4 cookies	130	18	6	1½
Thin Mints	4 cookies	140	18	10	2½
Upside-Downs	3 cookies	170	24	11	2¾
Golden Fruit					
All flavors	2 cookies	160	15	14	3½
Handi-Snack					
Cookie Jammers & Fruit Spread	1 pkg	130	26	14	3½
Health Valley					
Biscotti, all flavors	3 cookies	180	36	12	3
Cobbler Bites, all flavors	3 cookies	150	31	15	3¾

FOOD	SERVING SIZE	CALORIES	CARBO-HYDRATES (GRAMS)	SUGAR (GRAMS)	SUGAR (TSPS)
Health Valley (continued)					
Fat Free, all flavors	3 cookies	100	24	10–11	2½–2¾
Fat-Free Jumbo, all flavors	1 cookie	80	19	9	2¼
Wheat-Free, Dairy-Free Chocolate Chip	1 cookie	100	19	9	2¼
Heyday					
All varieties	1 cookie	110	13	11	2¾
Honey Maid					
Cinnamon Grahams	10 cookies	140	26	11	2¾
Honey Grahams	8 cookies	120	5	8	2
Oatmeal Crunch	8 cookies	130	23	8	2
Hydrox					
Original	3 cookies	150	21	11	2¾
Reduced fat	3 cookies	130	24	12	3
Keebler					
Animal Crackers, all varieties	6 cookies	130–150	18–24	9–10	2¼–2½
Animal Crackers, snack-size	1 pkg	250	41	14	3½
Butter	10 cookies	300	44	12	3
Chips Deluxe, all varieties	2 cookies	160–180	18–22	8–10	2–2½
Chocolate Lovers Chips Deluxe, snack-size	1 pkg	280	36	20	5
Classic Collection, all varieties	2 cookies	160	24	12	3
Cookie Stix	5 cookies	130–160	19–23	8–9	2–2¼
Country-Style Oatmeal	2 cookies	120	17	8	2
Danish Wedding	4 cookies	120	20	11	2¾
Droxies	3 cookies	140	21	12	3
Droxies, reduced fat	3 cookies	140	23	13	3¼
Elf Grahams, all varieties	8 cookies	130–140	23–24	7–9	1¾–2¼

FOOD	SERVING SIZE	CALORIES	CARBO-HYDRATES (GRAMS)	SUGAR (GRAMS)	SUGAR (TSPS)
Keebler (continued)					
Elf Grahams, reduced fat, all varieties	8 cookies	110–120	23–25	9–10	2¼–2½
E.L. Fudge, all varieties	3 cookies	180	24–27	11	2¾
Ernie's Animal Crackers	1 box	250	41	14	3½
Frosted Animal Crackers, snack-size	1 pkg	290	38	28	7
Fudge Shoppe Double Fudge n' Caramel	2 cookies	140	20	12	3
Fudge Shoppe Fudge Stripes	3 cookies	160	21	10	2½
Fudge Shoppe Fudge Stripes, reduced fat	3 cookies	140	21	12	3
Fudge Shoppe Fudge Sticks	3 cookies	150	20	15	3¾
Fudge Shoppe Grasshoppers	1 cookie	150	20	12	3
Fudge Shoppe Peanut Caramel Clusters	2 cookies	200	24	12	3
Ginger Snaps	5 cookies	150	24	10	2½
Golden Fruit Raisin Biscuits	2 cookies	160	30	18	4½
Golden Vanilla	8 cookies	150	20	9	2¼
Golden Vanilla, reduced fat	8 cookies	130	25	11	2¾
Lemon Coolers	5 cookies	140	21	10	2½
Lemon-Flavored Creme Sugar Wafers	3 cookies	130	19	14	3½
Mini Fudge Stripes, snack-size	1 pkg	280	38	16	4
Peanut Butter Creme Sugar Wafers	4 cookies	160	18	11	2¾
Rainbow Chips Deluxe, snack-size	1 pkg	290	36	18	4½

FOOD	SERVING SIZE	CALORIES	CARBO-HYDRATES (GRAMS)	SUGAR (GRAMS)	SUGAR (TSPS)
Keebler (continued)					
Shortbread w/Pecans Sandies, snack-size	1 pkg	300	33	13	3¼
Snackin' Grahams	21 cookies	130	23	9	2¼
Soft Batch, all varieties	2 cookies	140–160	20	10	2½
Soft Batch Homestyle Chocolate Chunk	2 cookies	260	34	20	5
Soft Batch Homestyle Double Chocolate Chunk	2 cookies	260	34	18	4½
Soft Batch Homestyle Oatmeal Raisin	2 cookies	260	40	22	5½
Sugar Wafers Cream Filled	3 cookies	130	19	14	3½
Sugar Wafers Lemon Filled	3 cookies	130	19	14	3½
Sugar Waffers Peanut Creme	4 cookies	160	18	11	3¾
Sugar Waffers Chocolate Creme	3 cookies	140	18	12	3
Vienna Fingers, all varieties	2 cookies	130–140	21	8–9	2–2½
Little Debbie					
Caramel Cookie Bars	1 pkg	160	23	17	4¼
Chocolate Chip Chewy	1 pkg	370	47	25	6¼
Chocolate Chip Crisp	1 pkg	210	26	10	2½
Creme Filled Chocolate	1 pkg (1.2 oz)	180	24	13	3¼
Easter Puffs	1 pkg	140	25	22	5½
Figaroos	1 pkg (1.2 oz)	160	31	22	5½
Figaroos	1 pkg (2 oz)	200	40	30	7½
Fudge Macaroons	1 pkg	140	18	13	3¼
Nutty Bars	1 bar	310	32	20	5
Oatmeal Crisp	1 pkg	210	27	14	3½

FOOD	SERVING SIZE	CALORIES	CARBO-HYDRATES (GRAMS)	SUGAR (GRAMS)	SUGAR (TSPS)
Little Debbie (continued)					
Oatmeal Lights	1 pkg	140	28	15	3¾
Oatmeal Raisin	1 pkg	320	50	29	7¼
Peanut Butter	1 pkg	210	27	15	3¾
Peanut Butter & Jelly Sandwich	1 pkg	130	22	14	3½
Peanut Butter Bars	1 pkg	270	33	20	5
Peanut Clusters	1 pkg	190	23	17	4¼
Pecan Shortbread	1 pkg	220	26	13	3¼
Snacks Nutty Bars Wafers w/Peanut Butter	2 bars	310	32	20	5
Snacks Oatmeal Creme Pies	1 pie	170	26	14	3½
Lorna Doone					
Cookies, all varieties	8 cookies	280	38	12	3
Lu					
Lu Chocolatiers	4 cookies	170	20	10	2½
Lu Chocolatiers Dipped	3 cookies	170	17	10	2½
Lu Le Petit Ecolier Dark Chocolate	2 cookies	130	17	9	2¼
Lu Little Schoolboy Mild Chocolate	2 cookies	130	15	8	2
Lu Marie Lu	6 cookies	340	50	12	3
Lu Truffle Lu	4 cookies	180	18	15	3¾
Mallopuffs					
Macaroons Chocolate	2 cookies	140	24	12	3
Mother's					
Butter	5 cookies	140	21	9	2¼
Checkerboard Wafers	8 cookies	150	20	10	2½
Chocolate Chip	2 cookies	160	20	11	2¾
Chocolate Chip Angel	3 cookies	180	21	8	2

FOOD	SERVING SIZE	CALORIES	CARBO-HYDRATES (GRAMS)	SUGAR (GRAMS)	SUGAR (TSPS)
Mother's (continued)					
Chocolate Chip Parade	4 cookies	130	19	8	2
Circus Animals	6 cookies	140	20	12	3
Cookie Parade	4 cookies	140	18	9	2¼
Dinosaur Grahams	2 cookies	130	24	12	3
Double Fudge	3 cookies	170	22	11	2¾
Duplex Creme	3 cookies	170	23	12	3
English Tea	2 cookies	180	26	12	3
Fig Bar	2 cookies	130	24	11	2¾
Fig Bar, fat free	2 cookies	140	32	18	4½
Fig Bar, whole wheat	2 cookies	130	20	12	3
Fig Bar, whole wheat, fat free	2 cookies	140	34	24	6
Flaky Flix Fudge	2 cookies	140	17	12	3
Flaky Flix Vanilla	2 cookies	140	17	14	3½
Frosted Holiday	4 cookies	130	19	11	2¾
Fudge Bowl Crowns	2 cookies	140	21	12	3
Fudge Bowl Nuggets	2 cookies	140	21	12	3
Iced Oatmeal	2 cookies	120	20	10	2½
Iced Oatmeal Bag	4 cookies	120	20	10	2½
Iced Raisin	2 cookies	180	24	12	3
MLB Double Header Duplex	3 cookies	170	23	12	3
Macaroon	2 cookies	150	18	8	2
Maries	3 cookies	170	28	9	2¼
North Poles	2 cookies	140	17	15	3¾
Oatmeal	2 cookies	110	17	14	3½
Oatmeal Chocolate Chip	2 cookies	120	19	9	2¼

FOOD	SERVING SIZE	CALORIES	CARBO-HYDRATES (GRAMS)	SUGAR (GRAMS)	SUGAR (TSPS)
Mother's (continued)					
Oatmeal Raisin	5 cookies	150	20	9	2¼
Oatmeal Walnut Chocolate Chip	2 cookies	130	17	9	2¼
Pecan Goldens	2 cookies	170	17	9	2¼
Rainbow Wafers	8 cookies	150	20	10	2½
Striped Shortbread	3 cookies	170	22	8	2
Sugar	2 cookies	170	19	8	2
Taffy	2 cookies	180	25	11	2¾
Triplet Assortment	2 cookies	140	18	11	2¾
Vanilla Wafers	6 cookies	150	24	14	3½
Walnut Fudge	4 cookies	260	32	14	3½
Mystic					
Mint	2 cookies	180	22	16	4
Nabisco					
Brown Edge Wafers	5 cookies	140	21	10	2½
Bugs Bunny Chocolate Graham	13 cookies	140	22	9	2¼
Bugs Bunny Cinnamon Graham	13 cookies	140	23	8	2
Cameo	2 cookies	130	21	10	2½
Chocolate Grahams	3 cookies	160	21	12	3
Chocolate Chip Snaps	7 cookies	150	24	10	2½
Chocolate Snaps	7 cookies	140	23	9	2¼
Danish Imported	5 cookies	170	22	8	2
Family Favorites Fudge Covered Grahams	3 cookies	140	19	10	2½
Family Favorites Fudge Striped Shortbread	3 cookies	160	22	11	2¾
Family Favorites Oatmeal	2 cookies	160	24	10	2½

FOOD	SERVING SIZE	CALORIES	CARBO-HYDRATES (GRAMS)	SUGAR (GRAMS)	SUGAR (TSPS)
Nabisco (continued)					
Family Favorites Vanilla Sandwich	3 cookies	170	25	12	3
Famous Chocolate Wafers	5 cookies	140	24	11	2¾
Ginger Snaps Old Fashioned	4 cookies	120	22	10	2½
Grahams	8 cookies	120	22	7	1¾
Marshmallow Puffs	1 cookie	90	14	11	2¾
Marshmallow Twirls	1 cookie	130	20	15	3¾
Newtons					
Apple, fat free	2 cookies	100	24	14	3½
Cranberry, fat free	2 cookies	100	23	15	3¾
Fig	2 cookies	110	20	13	3¼
Fig, fat free	1 cookie	100	22	15	3¾
Raspberry, fat free	2 cookies	100	23	14	3½
Strawberry, fat free	2 cookies	100	23	16	4
Nilla Wafers	8 cookies	140	24	12	3
Nutter Butter					
Bites Peanut Butter Sandwich	10 cookies	150	20	10	2½
Peanut Butter Sandwich	2 cookies	130	19	8	2
Peanut Creme Patties	5 cookies	160	17	8	2
Oreos					
Fudge-Covered Oreo	2 cookies	220	28	20	5
Halloween Treats Oreo	2 cookies	140	19	13	3¼
Oreo Double Stuf	2 cookies	140	19	12	3
Oreo Original	3 cookies	160	23	13	3¼
Reduced Fat Oreo	3 cookies	140	24	13	3¼
White Fudge Covered Oreo	2 cookies	220	28	20	5

FOOD	SERVING SIZE	CALORIES	CARBO-HYDRATES (GRAMS)	SUGAR (GRAMS)	SUGAR (TSPS)
Nabisco (continued)					
Pinwheels	1 cookie	130	21	16	4
SnackWell's					
Chocolate Chip Bite Size	13 cookies	130	22	10	2½
Chocolate Sandwich w/Chocolate Creme, reduced fat	4 cookies	200	40	22	5½
Devil's Food Cookie Cakes	2 cookies	100	24	14	3½
Golden Devil's Food Cookie Cakes	2 cookies	100	24	16	4
Mint Cream Sandwich	2 cookies	110	19	14	3½
Oatmeal Raisin	4 cookies	220	40	20	5
Vanilla Creme Sandwiches	2 cookies	110	21	10	2½
Newman's Own					
Fig Newman's Organic	2 cookies	120	28	15	3¾
Pepperidge Farm					
Bordeaux	4 cookies	130	19	12	3
Brussels	3 cookies	150	20	11	2¾
Chesapeake Chocolate Chunk Pecan	2 cookies	280	30	14	3½
Distinctive Selection	3 cookies	150	18	9	2¼
Geneva	3 cookies	160	19	8	2
Milano	3 cookies	180	21	11	2¾
Milano Double Chocolate	2 cookies	140	17	11	2¾
Milk Chocolate Milant	3 cookies	170	21	13	3¼
Mint Milano & Orange Milano	3 cookies	130	16	8	2
Nantucket Chocolate Chunk	1 cookie	140	16	9	2¼
Old Fashioned Gingerman	2 cookies	130	21	11	2¾

FOOD	SERVING SIZE	CALORIES	CARBO-HYDRATES (GRAMS)	SUGAR (GRAMS)	SUGAR (TSPS)
Pepperidge Farm (continued)					
Raspberry Tart	2 cookies	120	23	11	3¾
Sausalito Milk Chocolate & Macadamia Chocolate Chunk Cookies	1 cookie	140	16	9	2¼
Soft Bake Chocolate Chunk	1 cookie	130	16	9	2¼
Soft Bake Oatmeal Raisin	1 cookie	110	17	9	2¼
Sargento MooTown Snackers					
All flavors	1 pkg	140	19–20	11–12	2¾–3
Stella D'Oro					
Almond Toast	2 pieces	110	21	10	2¼
Anginette	4 pieces	140	23	17	4¼
Anisette Sponge	2 pieces	90	19	9	2¼
Anisette Toast	3 pieces	130	27	17	4¼
Breakfast Treats, chocolate	2 pieces	200	30	14	3½
Breakfast Treats, plain	2 pieces	200	32	14	3½
Chinese Dessert	1 piece	170	21	8	2
Como Delight	1 piece	140	18	8	2
Egg Jumbo	2 pieces	90	18	9	2¼
Indulgente Cashew Biscottini	1 piece	150	19	8	2
Lady Stella Assortment	3 pieces	130	19	8	2
Margherite Combination	2 pieces	140	22	9	2¼
Margherite	2 pieces	140	22	8	2
Sesame	3 pieces	150	21	8	2
Swiss Fudge	2 pieces	130	17	10	2¼
Sunshine					
Almond Crescents	4 pieces	150	22	10	2½
Animal Crackers	1 box	260	43	13	3¼

FOOD	SERVING SIZE	CALORIES	CARBO-HYDRATES (GRAMS)	SUGAR (GRAMS)	SUGAR (TSPS)
Sunshine (continued)					
Animal Crackers	14 crackers	140	24	7	1¾
Classics Chocolate Chips w/ Pecans	2 cookies	220	22	10	2½
Classics Chocolate Chips w/ Walnuts	2 cookies	200	22	12	3
Classics Premier Chocolate Chip	2 cookies	200	26	24	6
Dixie Vanilla	4 cookies	240	38	12	3
Fig Bars	2 cookies	110	20	11	2¾
Fudge Family Bears Vanilla	2 cookies	140	20	10	2½
Fudge Mint Patties	2 cookies	130	16	10	2½
Fudge Striped Shortbread	3 cookies	160	20	9	2¼
Ginger Snaps	7 cookies	130	22	9	2¼
Grahams Cinnamon	2 cookies	140	22	8	2
Grahams Fudge Dipped	4 cookies	170	21	11	2¾
Grahams Honey	2 cookies	120	20	6	1½
Grahamy Bears	1 pkg	260	41	11	2¾
Grahamy Bears	10 cookies	140	22	6	2½
Iced Gingerbread	5 cookies	130	19	6	1½
Iced Oatmeal	2 cookies	120	18	9	2¼
Jingles	6 cookies	150	22	9	2¼
Lemon Coolers	5 cookies	140	22	10	2½
Mini Chocolate Chip	5 cookies	160	20	8	2
Mini Fudge Royals	15 cookies	160	20	8	2
Oatmeal Chocolate Chip	3 cookies	170	23	11	2¾
Oatmeal Country Style	3 cookies	170	24	10	2½
School House	20 cookies	140	23	7	1¾

FOOD	SERVING SIZE	CALORIES	CARBO-HYDRATES (GRAMS)	SUGAR (GRAMS)	SUGAR (TSPS)
Sunshine (continued)					
Sugar Wafers Chocolate	3 cookies	130	17	11	2¾
Sugar Wafers Peanut Butter	4 cookies	170	19	10	2½
Sugar Wafers Vanilla	3 cookies	130	18	13	3¼
Tru Blu, all flavors	2 cookies	160	22	8	2
Vanilla Wafers	7 cookies	150	20	10	2½
Vienna Fingers	2 cookies	140	21	8	2
Vienna Fingers, low fat	2 cookies	130	23	10	2½
Tastykake					
Boxed Chocolate Chip	3 cookies	130	15	12	3
Boxed Oatmeal	3 cookies	130	14	7	1¾
Boxed Sugar Cookies	3 cookies	120	12	6	1½
Chocolate Chip Bar	1 bar	270	28	22	5½
Fudge Bar	1 bar	250	35	21	5¼
Oatmeal Raisin Bar	1 bar	260	32	18	4½
Teddy Grahams					
All flavors	24 pieces	140	22–23	8–9	2–2¼
Tree of Life					
Creme Supremes	2 cookies	120	18	10	2½
Creme Supremes Mint	2 cookies	120	18	10	2½
Fat Free, all flavors	2 cookies	120–140	28–32	6–7	1½–1¾
Fruit Bars Apple Spice	2 bars	120	22	9	2¼
Fruit Bars Fat Free Fig	2 bars	140	32	22	5½
Fruit Bars Fat Free Peach Apricot	2 bars	140	34	18	4½
Fruit Bars Fat Free Wildberry	2 bars	140	32	14	3½
Fruit Bars Fig	2 bars	120	21	10	2½
Honey-Sweet Colossal Carrot Cake	2 pieces	220	32	10	2½

FOOD	SERVING SIZE	CALORIES	CARBO-HYDRATES (GRAMS)	SUGAR (GRAMS)	SUGAR (TSPS)
Tree of Life (continued)					
Honey-Sweet Lemon Burst	2 cookies	220	30	10	2½
Honey-Sweet Oh-So-Oatmeal	2 cookies	220	28	8	2
Honey-Sweet Pecans-A-Plenty	2 cookies	250	28	8	2
Monster Fat Free Carrot Cake	½ cake	120	15	10	2½
Monster Fat Free Devil's Food Chocolate	½ cake	160	40	24	6
Monster Fat Free Maple Pecan	½ cake	180	40	20	5
Royal Vanilla	2 cookies	120	17	10	2½
Small World Animal Grahams	14 pieces	240	41	12	3
Small World Chocolate Chip	14 pieces	240	40	12	3
Soft-Bake Chocolate Chip	2 cookies	250	30	10	2½
Soft-Bake Double Fudge	2 cookies	220	32	10	2½
Soft-Bake Maui Macaroon	2 cookies	270	24	8	2
Soft-Bake Oatmeal	2 cookies	230	32	10	2½
Soft-Bake Peanut Butter	2 cookies	250	26	8	2
Wheat-Free California Carob	2 cookies	210	28	8	2
Wheat-Free Mountain Maple Walnut	2 cookies	200	18	8	2
Walkers					
Shortbread Triangles	4 cookies	200	24	8	2
Weight Watchers					
Apple Raisin Bar	2 bars	140	28	8	2
Chocolate Chip	2 cookies	140	22	15	3¾
Chocolate Sandwich	2 sandwiches	140	23	16	4

FOOD	SERVING SIZE	CALORIES	CARBO-HYDRATES (GRAMS)	SUGAR (GRAMS)	SUGAR (TSPS)
Weight Watchers (continued)					
Fruit Filled Fig	2 cookies	170	32	18	4½
Fruit Filled Raspberry	2 cookies	140	32	14	3½
Oatmeal Raisin	2 cookies	120	22	13	3¼

Donuts

Ready to Eat

FOOD	SERVING SIZE	CALORIES	CARBO-HYDRATES (GRAMS)	SUGAR (GRAMS)	SUGAR (TSPS)
Country Hearth					
Plain	1 donut	150	19	11	2¾
Sugared-coated	1 donut	160	22	15	3¾
Dutch Mill					
Cider	1 donut	240	35	23	5¾
Cinnamon	1 donut	210	26	12	3
Donut Holes Double-Dipped Chocolate	6 holes	440	38	10	2½
Donut Holes Shootin' Stars	3 holes	190	23	12	3
Double-Dipped Chocolate	1 donut	180	31	9	2¼
Glazed	1 donut	250	34	23	5¾
Glazed Chocolate	1 donut	270	40	10	2½
Plain	1 donut	210	25	9	2¼
Sugared-coated	1 donut	220	27	12	3
Entenmann's					
Country Powdered	1 donut	240	24	12	3
Crumb	1 donut	260	34	20	5
Donut Holes	4 holes	200	29	18	4½
Glazed Butternut	1 donut	270	35	21	5¼
Rich Frosted Chocolate	1 donut	290	27	15	3¾
Freihofer's					
Assorted	1 donut	270	26	15	3¾

FOOD	SERVING SIZE	CALORIES	CARBO-HYDRATES (GRAMS)	SUGAR (GRAMS)	SUGAR (TSPS)
Hostess					
Assorted	1 donut	200	23	14	3½
Cinnamon Family Pack	1 donut	110	15	8	2
Cinnamon Swirl	1 donut	180	28	10	2½
Crumb Regular	1 donut	130	14	8	2
Frosted Regular	1 donut	180	20	12	3
Gem Donettes Cinnamon	6 donettes	320	53	28	7
Gem Donettes Frosted	6 donettes	390	42	21	5¼
Gem Donnettes Frosted Strawberry Filled	3 donettes	240	29	15	3¾
Gem Donettes Powdered	6 donettes	350	47	23	5¾
Gem Donettes Powdered Strawberry Filled	3 donettes	210	31	15	3¾
Glazed Party	1 donut	260	39	14	3½
Jumbo Frosted	1 donut	260	28	14	3½
Jumbo Plain	1 donut	140	16	8	2
Jumbo Powdered	1 donut	160	19	11	2¾
O's Raspberry Filled Powdered	1 donut	230	35	17	4¼
Old Fashioned Glazed	1 donut	250	33	15	3¾
Old Fashioned Glazed Honey Wheat	1 donut	250	33	15	3¾
Old Fashioned Plain	1 donut	170	21	9	2¼
Plain Regular	1 donut	120	13	8	2
Powdered Family Pack	1 donut	110	15	8	2
Little Debbie					
Donut Sticks	1 pkg (1.6 oz)	210	25	14	3½
Donut Sticks	1 pkg (2 oz)	250	30	17	4¼
Donut Sticks	1 pkg (2.5 oz)	320	37	21	5¼
Donut Sticks	1 pkg (3 oz)	390	45	26	6½

FOOD	SERVING SIZE	CALORIES	CARBO-HYDRATES (GRAMS)	SUGAR (GRAMS)	SUGAR (TSPS)

English Muffins

English muffins contain approximately 2 to 3 teaspoons of sugar unless raisins or other fruit is added. In that case, they contain approximately 3 to 4 teaspoons of sugar per muffin. See also Muffins.

Muffins

See also English Muffins.

Frozen

FOOD	SERVING SIZE	CALORIES	CARBO-HYDRATES (GRAMS)	SUGAR (GRAMS)	SUGAR (TSPS)
Pepperidge Farm					
Apple Cinnamon	2 oz	160	28	11	2¾
Sara Lee					
Blueberry	1 muffin	220	27	12	3
Corn	1 muffin	260	30	14	3½
Weight Watchers					
Blueberry	1 muffin	160	38	15	3¾
Banana	1 muffin	170	41	17	4¼
Chocolate Chocolate Chip	1 muffin	190	39	14	3½

Mixes

FOOD	SERVING SIZE	CALORIES	CARBO-HYDRATES (GRAMS)	SUGAR (GRAMS)	SUGAR (TSPS)
Betty Crocker					
Banana Nut	3 tbs dry mix	170	24	12	3
Double Chocolate	¼ cup dry mix	200	25	13	3¼
Lemon Poppy Seed	¼ cup dry mix	190	30	16	4
Twice Blueberry	¼ cup dry mix	140	25	13	3¼
Betty Crocker Sweet Rewards (low fat)					
Apple Cinnamon	¼ cup dry mix	140	30	18	4½
Wild Blueberry	3 tbs dry mix	130	27	15	3¾

FOOD	SERVING SIZE	CALORIES	CARBO-HYDRATES (GRAMS)	SUGAR (GRAMS)	SUGAR (TSPS)
Duncan Hines					
Blueberry	1/12 pkg	190	30	17	4¼
Cinnamon Swirl	1/12 pkg	190	33	19	4¾
Cranberry Orange Premium	1/12 pkg	150	26	13	3¼
Jiffy					
Apple Cinnamon, as prepared	1 muffin	190	28	13	3¼
Banana Nut, as prepared	1 muffin	180	25	11	2¾
Blueberry, as prepared	1 muffin	190	28	13	3¼
Bran w/ Dates, as prepared	1 muffin	170	26	12	3
Corn, as prepared	1 muffin	180	26	8	2
Honey Date, as prepared	1 muffin	170	27	11	2¾
Oatmeal, as prepared	1 muffin	180	26	10	2½
Krusteaz					
Almond Poppyseed	4 oz	425	54	39	9¾
Apple Cinnamon, low fat	2 oz	141	31	18	4½
Banana Nut	2 oz	191	29	14	3½
Blackberry	4 oz	420	51	35	8¾
Blueberry	2 oz	171	30	18	4½
Blueberry, low fat	2 oz	131	29	19	4¾
Honey Bran	2 oz	171	29	13	3¼
Oat Bran	2 oz	161	32	14	3½
Orange Raisin	2 oz	171	31	14	3½
Plain	2 oz	181	31	17	4¼
Plain, low fat	2 oz	151	32	21	5¼
Whole Wheat, low fat	2 oz	151	32	19	4¾
Pillsbury					
Apple Cinnamon	⅓ cup	180	31	18	4½
Banana Nut	¼ cup	170	27	14	3½

FOOD	SERVING SIZE	CALORIES	CARBO-HYDRATES (GRAMS)	SUGAR (GRAMS)	SUGAR (TSPS)
Pillsbury (continued)					
Blueberry	⅓ cup	180	31	18	4½
Blueberry, low fat	¼ cup	150	31	19	4¾
Chocolate Chip	⅓ cup	190	31	18	4½
Cinnamon	¼ cup	160	27	15	3¾
Strawberry	⅓ cup	180	31	18	4½
Wildberry	⅓ cup	180	31	18	4½

Ready to Eat

FOOD	SERVING SIZE	CALORIES	CARBO-HYDRATES (GRAMS)	SUGAR (GRAMS)	SUGAR (TSPS)
Dutch Mill					
Apple Oat Bran	1 muffin	180	31	15	3¾
Banana Walnut	1 muffin	220	33	15	3¾
Carrot	1 muffin	190	31	19	4¾
Corn	1 muffin	190	31	14	3½
Cranberry Orange	1 muffin	170	26	14	3½
Raisin Bran	1 muffin	230	37	12	3
Entenmann's					
Banana Crunch	2 oz	220	32	18	4½
Little Bites Blueberry	4 bites	190	26	16	4
Cinnamon Apple, fat free	2 oz	130	29	16	4
French Crumb	2 oz	210	29	15	3¾
Sweet Roll, Blueberry Cheese, fat free	2.4 oz	140	31	18	4½
Sweet Roll, Cinnamon Raisin, fat free	2.2 oz	160	36	20	5
Freihofer's					
Corn Toasters	1 muffin	130	18	7	1¾
Hostess					
Mini, all varieties	5 muffins	240–260	28–30	14–15	3½–3¾
Muffin Loaf Blueberry	1 muffin	440	62	34	8½

FOOD	SERVING SIZE	CALORIES	CARBO-HYDRATES (GRAMS)	SUGAR (GRAMS)	SUGAR (TSPS)
Hostess (continued)					
Oat Bran	1 muffin	160	22	10	2½
Oat Bran Banana Nut	1 muffin	150	22	9	2¼
Otis Spunkmeyer					
Chocolate Chocolate Chip	1 muffin	210	41	26	6½

Pancakes

In general, there are between 1¾ and 2½ teaspoons of sugar per serving of pancakes based on three medium pancakes or one-third cup of dry mix. Frozen, packaged pancakes that are prepared in the microwave usually have between 3 and 4 teaspoons of sugar per serving. Read labels. Don't forget to take into account the sugar content of the syrup! See Pancake and Waffle Syrup under Sweeteners and Toppings on page 162.

Pies

Generic

FOOD	SERVING SIZE	CALORIES	CARBO-HYDRATES (GRAMS)	SUGAR (GRAMS)	SUGAR (TSPS)
Apple	⅛ of 9" pie	296	43	22	5½
Blackberry	⅛ of 9" pie	400	56	23	5¾
Blueberry	⅛ of 9" pie	400	49	20	5
Cheesecake	2.5 oz	257	20	18	4½
Cherry	⅛ of 9" pie	486	69	30	7½
Chocolate cream	⅛ of 8" pie	340	37	29	7¾
Coconut custard	⅛ of 9" pie	270	32	19	4¾
Fruit Pie, fried	1 pie	404	54	15	3¾
Lemon meringue	⅛ of 9" pie	369	50	33	8¼
Mince	⅛ of 9" pie	474	57	18	4½
Peach	⅛ of 9" pie	375	55	35	8¾
Pecan pie	⅛ of 9" pie	503	64	58	14½

FOOD	SERVING SIZE	CALORIES	CARBO-HYDRATES (GRAMS)	SUGAR (GRAMS)	SUGAR (TSPS)
Generic (continued)					
Pumpkin	⅛ of 9" pie	316	41	29	7¼
Frozen					
Banquet					
Apple	⅕ pie	300	41	22	5½
Banana Cream	⅓ pie	350	39	28	7
Cherry	⅕ pie	290	39	14	3½
Chocolate Cream	⅓ pie	360	43	33	8¼
Coconut Cream	⅓ pie	350	39	30	7½
Lemon Cream	⅓ pie	360	43	31	7¾
Mincemeat	⅕ pie	310	46	26	6½
Peach	⅕ pie	260	36	17	4¼
Pumpkin	⅕ pie	250	40	21	5¼
Kineret					
Apple Homestyle	⅙ pie	313	41	20	5
Mrs. Smith					
Apple	⅙ of 8" pie	270	41	20	5
Apple	⅛ of 9" pie	370	50	27	6¾
Apple	⅒ of 10" pie	280	43	22	5½
Apple Cranberry	⅙ of 8" pie	280	43	22	5½
Apple Lattice, ready to serve	⅙ of 8" pie	310	45	23	5¾
Banana Cream	¼ of 8" pie	250	40	28	7
Berry	⅙ of 8" pie	280	44	22	5½
Blackberry	⅙ of 8" pie	280	43	21	5¼
Blueberry	⅙ of 8" pie	260	39	17	4¼
Boston Cream	⅛ of 8" pie	170	29	19	4¾
Cherry	⅙ of 8" pie	270	41	19	4¾

FOOD	SERVING SIZE	CALORIES	CARBO-HYDRATES (GRAMS)	SUGAR (GRAMS)	SUGAR (TSPS)
Mrs. Smith (continued)					
Cherry	⅛ of 9″ pie	320	48	24	6
Cherry Lattice, ready to serve	⅕ of 8″ pie	320	47	22	5½
Chocolate Cream	¼ of 8″ pie	290	37	25	6¼
Coconut Cream	¼ of 8″ pie	280	36	25	6¼
Coconut Custard	⅕ of 8″ pie	280	35	18	4½
Dutch Apple	⅒ of 10″ pie	320	50	23	5¾
Dutch Apple	⅙ of 8″ pie	310	48	21	5¼
Dutch Apple	⅑ of 9″ pie	300	48	27	6¾
French Silk Cream	⅕ of 0″ pie	410	55	42	10½
Hearty Pumpkin	⅕ of 8″ pie	280	46	26	6½
Lemon Cream	¼ of 8″ pie	270	36	25	6¼
Lemon Meringue	⅕ of 8″ pie	300	54	37	9¼
Mince	⅙ of 8″ pie	300	48	23	5¾
Peach	⅙ of 8″ pie	260	37	17	4¼
Peach	⅛ of 9″ pie	310	46	25	6¼
Pecan	⅛ of 10″ pie	500	68	40	10
Pumpkin	⅛ of 10″ pie	250	42	24	6
Pumpkin	⅕ of 8″ pie	270	44	24	6
Red Raspberry	⅙ of 8″ pie	280	43	21	5¼
Strawberry Rhubarb	⅕ of 8″ pie	520	73	45	11¼
Strawberry Rhubarb	⅙ of 8″ pie	280	44	22	5½
Sweet potato	⅙ of 8″ pie	280	43	22	5½
Sara Lee					
Chocolate Silk	⅛ pie	500	49	35	8¾
Coconut Cream	⅛ pie	480	47	35	8¾
Fruits of the Forest	⅛ pie	340	40	15	3¾

FOOD	SERVING SIZE	CALORIES	CARBO-HYDRATES (GRAMS)	SUGAR (GRAMS)	SUGAR (TSPS)
Sara Lee (continued)					
Homestyle Mince	⅛ pie	390	56	30	7½
Homestyle Pecan	⅛ pie	520	70	28	7
Homestyle Pumpkin	⅛ pie	260	37	18	4½
Homestyle Raspberry	⅛ pie	380	48	20	5
Homestyle, all other fruit varieties	⅛ pie	330–360	26–30	26–30	6½–7½
Lemon Meringue	⅛ pie	350	59	42	10½
Slice Lemon Icebox	1 pie	260	41	37	9½
Slice Southern Pecan	1 pie	470	62	31	7¾
Weight Watchers					
Chocolate Cream	2 oz	170	31	20	5
Mississippi Mud	2 oz	160	24	13	3¼

Mixes

FOOD	SERVING SIZE	CALORIES	CARBO-HYDRATES (GRAMS)	SUGAR (GRAMS)	SUGAR (TSPS)
Jell-O No Bake Desserts					
Cherry Cheesecake	⅛ pie	340	52	33	8½
Chocolate Silk Pie	⅙ pie	320	37	20	5
Double Layer Chocolate	⅛ pie	260	34	21	5¼
Double Layer Cookies & Cream	⅙ pie	390	51	32	8¾
Double Layer Lemon Dessert	⅛ pie	260	36	25	6¼
Homestyle Cheesecake	⅙ pie	360	50	35	7¾
Peanut Butter Cup	⅛ pie	380	41	28	7
Real Cheese	⅙ pie	360	47	33	8¼
Strawberry Cheesecake	⅛ pie	340	52	36	9
Strawberry Swirl Cheesecake, reduced fat	⅛ pie	250	44	33	8¼

FOOD	SERVING SIZE	CALORIES	CARBO-HYDRATES (GRAMS)	SUGAR (GRAMS)	SUGAR (TSPS)
Little Debbie					
Marshmallow Banana	1 pkg (1.4 oz)	160	27	17	4¼
Marshmallow Banana	1 pkg (2 oz)	240	40	25	6¼
Marshmallow Banana	1 pkg (2.7 oz)	320	54	33	8¼
Marshmallow Chocolate	1 pkg (1.4 oz)	160	27	16	4
Marshmallow Chocolate	1 pkg (2 oz)	240	40	24	6
Marshmallow Chocolate	1 pkg (2.7 oz)	320	53	32	8
Oatmeal Creme	1 pkg (1.3 oz)	170	25	16	4
Oatmeal Creme	1 pkg (3 oz)	360	58	36	9
Oatmeal Creme	1 pkg (2.5 oz)	300	48	30	7½
Raisin Creme	1 pkg (1.2 oz)	140	23	16	4
Raisin Creme	1 pkg (2.5 oz)	290	47	32	8

Pie Filling

See Puddings, Custards, and Pie Fillings under Desserts.

BEVERAGES

Alcoholic and Malt Drinks

FOOD	SERVING SIZE	CALORIES	CARBO-HYDRATES (GRAMS)	SUGAR (GRAMS)	SUGAR (TSPS)
Beer, regular	12 fl oz	150	13	13	3¼
Beer, lite	12 fl oz	95	5	5	1¼
Bloody Mary (tomato juice, vodka, and lemon juice)	10 fl oz	230	10	10	2½
Daiquiri (rum, lime juice, and sugar)	6.8 fl oz	259	33	33	8¼
Distilled spirits, all types, 80 proof	1.5 fl oz jigger	94–110	0	0	0

FOOD	SERVING SIZE	CALORIES	CARBO-HYDRATES (GRAMS)	SUGAR (GRAMS)	SUGAR (TSPS)
Gin and tonic (tonic water, gin, and lime juice)	7.5 fl oz	171	16	16	4
Liqueur, coffee, 53 proof	1.5 fl oz	175	24	24	6
Liqueur, coffee w/ cream, 34 proof	1.5 fl oz	154	10	10	2½
Malt beverage, nonalcoholic	12 fl oz	32	5	5	1¼
Pina colada (pineapple jce, rum, sugar, and coconut cream)	6.8 fl oz	526	61	61	15¼
Pina colada (pineapple jce, rum, sugar, and coconut cream)	4.5 fl oz	264	40	40	10
Screwdriver (orange jce and vodka)	7 fl oz	175	18	18	4½
Tequila sunrise	6.8 fl oz	232	24	24	6
Tequila sunrise (orange jce, tequila, lime jce, grenadine	5.5 fl oz	189	15	15	3¾
Tom Collins (club soda, gin, lemon jce, and sugar)	7.5 fl oz	122	3	3	¾
Whiskey sour (lemon jce, whiskey, and sugar)	3 fl oz	122	5	5	1¼
Whiskey sour, prep from bottled mix	2 fl oz mix 1.5 fl oz whiskey	158	14	14	3½
Whiskey sour, prep from powdered mix (17 g pkt)	1.5 fl oz whisky, 1.5 fl oz water	169	16	16	4
Whiskey sour, mix, bottled	2 fl oz	55	14	14	3½
Wine, dessert, sweet	2 fl oz	90	7	7	1¾
Wine, red	3½ fl oz	75	2	2	½
Wine, rose	3½ fl oz	73	1	1	¼
Wine, white	3½ fl oz	80	less than 1	less than 1	less than 1

FOOD	SERVING SIZE	CALORIES	CARBO-HYDRATES (GRAMS)	SUGAR (GRAMS)	SUGAR (TSPS)

Alcoholic Mixers

FOOD	SERVING SIZE	CALORIES	CARBO-HYDRATES (GRAMS)	SUGAR (GRAMS)	SUGAR (TSPS)
Bacardi					
Margarita Mix	8 fl oz	100	25	23	5¾
Pina Colada	8 fl oz	140	34	32	8
Rum Runner	8 fl oz	140	35	33	8¼
Strawberry Daiquiri	8 fl oz	140	35	33	8¼
Canada Dry					
Collins Mixer	8 fl oz	120	25	25	6¼
Lemon Sour	8 fl oz	100	21	21	5¼
Sour Mixer	8 fl oz	90	22	22	5½
Tonic Water	8 fl oz	100	24	24	6
Darby's					
Mocha Mudslide Cocktail Mix	4 oz	300	69	40	10
Jose Cuervo					
Strawberry Margarita Mix	4 oz	100	24	24	6
Mr. & Mrs. T					
Pina Colada Mix	4 oz	100	23	21	5¼
Sweet & Sour	4 oz	100	23	21	5¼
Sauza					
Margarita Mix	6 oz	140	34	34	8½
Schweppes					
Collins Mixer	8 fl oz	100	24	24	6
Lemon-Lime	8 fl oz	100	25	25	6¼
Tonic Water, all varieties	8 fl oz	90	20	20	5
Tabasco					
Blood Mary Mix	8.4 fl oz	56	11	8	2
Bloody Mary Mix Extra Spicy	8.4 fl oz	56	11	10	2½

FOOD	SERVING SIZE	CALORIES	CARBO-HYDRATES (GRAMS)	SUGAR (GRAMS)	SUGAR (TSPS)

Coffee

When calculating the amount of sugar you are consuming when you drink a cup of coffee, don't forget to include the sugar content of the milk or cream and the table sugar you may add. Coffeemate, which is often used instead of milk or cream also contains sugar. A serving size of 4 teaspoons for all varieties has approximately 50 calories, 15 grams of carbohydrates, 6–8 grams or 1½–2 teaspoons of sugar.

FOOD	SERVING SIZE	CALORIES	CARBO-HYDRATES (GRAMS)	SUGAR (GRAMS)	SUGAR (TSPS)
General Foods					
Café Vienna	1½ tsps	70	11	10	2½
International Flavored Instant Coffee, Prepared*, all varieties	8 oz	50–70	9–12	9–11	1¾–2¼
International Cappuccino Coolers	1 packet	60	14–15	14–15	3½–3¾
Maxwell House					
Café Cappuccino, all varieties	8 oz	90–100	17–19	16–18	4–4½
Iced Cappuccino	8 oz	140	27	24	6

Diet Drinks, Liquid Diets, and Nutritional Drinks

Whether a drink is a weight-loss product or a meal replacement, you'll find both types listed below.

Powder

FOOD	SERVING SIZE	CALORIES	CARBO-HYDRATES (GRAMS)	SUGAR (GRAMS)	SUGAR (TSPS)
Ensure					
Powder	½ c w/ ¾ c water	250	34	13	3¼

*Except Café Francais which has 1 teaspoon of sugar.

FOOD	SERVING SIZE	CALORIES	CARBO-HYDRATES (GRAMS)	SUGAR (GRAMS)	SUGAR (TSPS)
Slim Fast					
Chocolate, chocolate malt, strawberry, and vanilla	1 oz	100	20	17	4¼
Ultra-Slim Fast Powder, all flavors	1 oz	111–120	22–25	16–20	4–5
Ready to Drink					
Boost					
Nutritional Drink, Strawberry	8 fl oz	240	40	27	6¾
Nutritional Drink, Vanilla Flavored	8 fl oz	240	40	23	5¾
Ensure					
Fiber Nutrition Drink	8 fl oz	360	42	17	4¼
Butter Pecan Nutrition Drink	8 fl oz	250	40	14	3½
Chocolate Nutrition Drink	8 fl oz	250	40	18	4½
Chocolate Royal Nutrition Drink	8 fl oz	230	31	21	5¼
Strawberry Nutrition Drink	8 fl oz	250	40	15	3¾
Vanilla Nutrition Drink	8 fl oz	250	40	14	3½
Vanilla Nutrition Drink, lite	8 fl oz	200	33	18	4½
Ensure					
Ensure Plus Nutrition Drink, all varieties	8 fl oz	360	47	15–17	3¾–4¼
Nestlé					
Success Diet Drink Chocolate Mocha Supreme	10 fl oz	200	37	32	8
Success Diet Drink Creamy Milk Chocolate	10 fl oz	200	36	30	7½
Success Diet Drink Milk Chocolate Almond	10 fl oz	200	36	32	8

FOOD	SERVING SIZE	CALORIES	CARBO-HYDRATES (GRAMS)	SUGAR (GRAMS)	SUGAR (TSPS)
Nestlé (continued)					
Success Diet Drink Strawberries 'N Cream	10 fl oz	200	37	30	7½
Success Diet Drink Vanilla Delight	10 fl oz	200	38	33	8¼
Slim Fast					
Ultra-Slim Fast Diet Drink Chocolate Fudge	11 fl oz	220	42	34	8½
Ultra-Slim Fast Diet Drink Chocolate Royale	11 fl oz	220	38	33	8¼
Ultra-Slim Fast Diet Drink French Vanilla	11 fl oz	220	38	33	8¼
Ultra-Slim Fast Diet Drink Milk Chocolate	11 fl oz	220	42	35	8¾
Ultra-Slim Fast Diet Drink Strawberry Supreme,	11 fl oz	220	42	37	9¼
Ultra-Slim Fast Healthy Shake Vanilla	15 fl oz	100	20	18	4½
Ultra-Slim Fast Juice Base, apple cran raspberry	11.5 fl oz	220	48	43	10¾
Ultra-Slim Fast Juice Base, orange, strawberry, banana	11.5 fl oz	220	47	42	10½

Fruit-Flavored Drinks

Beware: All fruit-flavored drinks contain added sugar!

Powdered or Concentrated

FOOD	SERVING SIZE	CALORIES	CARBO-HYDRATES (GRAMS)	SUGAR (GRAMS)	SUGAR (TSPS)
Country Time					
Lemonade as prepared, all varieties	8 fl oz	70	17	17	4¼
Crystal Light, Iced, sweetened	8 fl oz	70	17	17	4¼

FOOD	SERVING SIZE	CALORIES	CARBO-HYDRATES (GRAMS)	SUGAR (GRAMS)	SUGAR (TSPS)
Country Time (continued)					
Kool-Aid mix, prep w/sugar and water	8 fl oz	100	25	25	6¼
Kool-Aid mix, sweetened	8 fl oz	60	16–17	16–17	4–4¼
Kraft, Country Time, Lemonade & Pink Lemonade	8 fl oz	70	17	17	4¼
Kraft, Country Time Lem'n Berry Sippers, all varieties	8 fl oz	90	21	21	5¼
Lipton					
Iced, w/ sugar and lemon	8 fl oz	90	22	22	5½
Mott's					
Apple Cranberry	2 fl oz	170	40	37	9¼
Apple Raspberry	2 fl oz	130	31	29	7¼
Mott's In A Minute, Fruit Punch & Grape Apple Drink	2 fl oz	140	34	32	8
Nestlé					
Strawberry Flavor	2 tbsp	90	22	21	5¼
Swiss Miss Apple Cider Mix	2 tbsp	84	20	19	4¾
Newman's Own					
Lemonade	8 fl oz	110	27	27	6¾
Tang					
All varieties	8 fl oz	90–100	23–25	23–25	5¾–6¼
Wyler's					
Lemonade	8 fl oz	78	20	20	5
Tropical Punch & Wild Strawberry	8 fl oz	85	21	21	5¼

Frozen

FOOD	SERVING SIZE	CALORIES	CARBO-HYDRATES (GRAMS)	SUGAR (GRAMS)	SUGAR (TSPS)
Minute Maid					
All lemonades	8 fl oz	80–120	29–30	28	7

FOOD	SERVING SIZE	CALORIES	CARBO-HYDRATES (GRAMS)	SUGAR (GRAMS)	SUGAR (TSPS)
Ready to Drink					
Betty Crocker					
Gushers Fruitomic Punch	1 pouch	90	20	12	3
Capri Sun					
All varieties	1 pouch	90–100	24–27	24–27	6–6¾
Country Time					
Lem'n Berry Sippers, All varieties	8 fl oz	90	21	21	5¼
Lemonade & Pink Lemonade	8 fl oz	70	17	17	4¼
Fruitopia					
Tropical Considerations	8 fl oz	75	19	18	4½
All other varieties	8 fl oz	110–127	28–32	27–30	6¾–7½
Gatorade					
All flavors	8 fl oz	50	14	14	3½
Hansen					
Juice Drink Energy Smoothie Island Blast	11.5 fl oz	170	42	42	10½
Juice Drink Fruit Smoothie Strawberry Banana	11.5 fl oz	120	31	31	7¾
Super Energy Smoothie Tropical Blast	11.5 fl oz	170	40	40	10
Super Power Smoothie Berry Splash	11.5 fl oz	170	41	40	10
Super Protein Smoothie Banana Citrus	11.5 fl oz	290	58	38	9½
Super Vita Orange Carrot Smoothie	11.5 fl oz	170	40	40	10
Kool-Aid					
Bursts, all brands	7 fl oz	100	24–25	24–25	6–6½
Splash, all brand	7 fl oz	110–120	29–31	29–31	7¼–7¾
Minute Maid					
Concord Punch	8 fl oz	127	32	31	7¾

FOOD	SERVING SIZE	CALORIES	CARBO-HYDRATES (GRAMS)	SUGAR (GRAMS)	SUGAR (TSPS)
Minute Maid (continued)					
Cranberry Apple Cocktail	8 fl oz	167	42	42	10
Cranberry, Apple, Raspberry Blend	8 fl oz	123	33	31	7¾
Five Alive	8 fl oz	123	31	29	7¼
Fruit Punch	8 fl oz	125	31	31	7¾
Fruit Punch	8 fl oz	114	30	29	7¼
Lemonade & Pink Lemonade	8 fl oz	110	28	26	6½
Lemonade Cranberry	8 fl oz	120	31	29	7¼
Lemonade Raspberry	8 fl oz	130	28	28	/
Mott's					
Lemonade	10 fl oz	160	41	35	8¾
Newman's					
Lemonade Carton	8 fl oz	110	27	27	6¾
Lemonade Glass	10 fl oz	140	34	34	8½
Lemonade Roadside Virginia	8 fl oz	110	27	27	6¾
Ocean Spray					
Cranapple	6 fl oz	130	32	32	8
Cranapple, Crangrape & Cranraspberry	6 fl oz	110	27	27	6¾
Crangrape	6 fl oz	110	26	26	6½
Cranraspberry	6 fl oz	110	27	27	6¾
Odwalla					
Lemonade Honey	8 fl oz	70	26	25	6¼
Lemonade Strawberry	8 fl oz	150	40	38	9½
Lemonade	1 can	140	40	40	10
Snapple					
All varieties	16 fl oz	110	29	27	6¾

FOOD	SERVING SIZE	CALORIES	CARBO-HYDRATES (GRAMS)	SUGAR (GRAMS)	SUGAR (TSPS)
Sunkist					
Fruit Punch	12 fl oz	180	49	49	12¼

Juice, Fruit

Ounce for ounce, there is approximately the same amount of sugar in fruit juice as there is in a soft drink. As mentioned under Fruit, it's always a good idea to eat your fruit whole. When serving fruit juice to children, water down juice to ⅕ fruit juice to ⅘ water. The brand-name juices listed under the Canned section may contain juices other than those mentioned, but they do not contain added sugar. In these products, the main ingredient is usually concentrated fruit juice. As for the juices listed below in the Frozen section, which are not brand-name products, they are usually 100% fruit juice, but most likely also come from concentrate. Once again, frozen fruit juice may contain fruit juice concentrate from juices that do not appear in the name of the juice. See also Fruit.

Fresh

FOOD	SERVING SIZE	CALORIES	CARBO-HYDRATES (GRAMS)	SUGAR (GRAMS)	SUGAR (TSPS)
Apple	8 fl oz	116	29	28	7
Grapefruit	8 fl oz	96	23	23	5¾
Orange	8 fl oz	112	26	25	6¼
Tangerine	8 fl oz	106	25	25	6¼

Canned

FOOD	SERVING SIZE	CALORIES	CARBO-HYDRATES (GRAMS)	SUGAR (GRAMS)	SUGAR (TSPS)
Ceres					
Apricot Blend	8 fl oz	120	30	29	7¼
Mango Blend	8 fl oz	120	27	20	6¾
Medley of Fruit Blend	8 fl oz	120	31	29	7¼
Papaya Blend	8 fl oz	120	30	27	6¾

FOOD	SERVING SIZE	CALORIES	CARBO-HYDRATES (GRAMS)	SUGAR (GRAMS)	SUGAR (TSPS)
Ceres (continued)					
Peach Blend	8 fl oz	120	29	24	6
Youngberry Blend	8 fl oz	120	30	25	6¼
Kern					
All Nectar Apple	11.5 fl oz	210	58	53	13¼
All Nectar Apricot	11.5 fl oz	220	52	44	11
All Nectar Apricot Mango	11.5 fl oz	210	51	48	12
All Nectar Guava	11.5 fl oz	220	54	47	11¾
All Nectar Mango	11.5 fl oz	210	52	45	11¼
All Nectar Peach Passion Fruit	11.5 fl oz	210	52	48	12
Libby's Concentrate					
Cherry	2 oz in 8 fl oz water	120	30	30	7½
Cranberry	2 oz in 8 fl oz water	130	33	30	7½
Mott's					
Apple cranberry	8 fl oz	120	30	24	6
Apple Grape	8 fl oz	130	33	31	7¾
Apple Raspberry	8 fl oz	120	31	28	7
Ocean Spray Concentrate					
CranApple	2 oz in 8 fl oz water	160	40	40	10
CranGrape	2 oz in 8 fl oz water	160	41	41	10¼
CranRaspberry	2 oz in 8 fl oz water	140	36	36	9
CranTangerine	2 oz in 8 fl oz water	150	38	38	9½
Welsh's					
Apple	2 oz in 8 fl oz water	120	29	28	7

FOOD	SERVING SIZE	CALORIES	CARBO-HYDRATES (GRAMS)	SUGAR (GRAMS)	SUGAR (TSPS)
Welsh's (continued)					
Concord Grape	2 oz in 8 fl oz water	130	33	32	8
Fruit Blend	2 oz in 8 fl oz water	130	32	30	7½
Tropical Passion	2 oz in 8 fl oz water	140	35	34	8½
Wild Berry	2 oz in 8 fl oz water	150	37	36	9
Frozen					
Grape	8 fl oz	130	32	30	7½
Grapefruit	8 fl oz	94	22	22	5½
Orange juice	8 fl oz	112	27	26	6½
Pineapple juice	8 fl oz	140	34	31	7¾
Raspberry juice	8 fl oz	120	29	29	7¼
White Grape juice	8 fl oz	170	42	40	10

Juice, Vegetable

FOOD	SERVING SIZE	CALORIES	CARBO-HYDRATES (GRAMS)	SUGAR (GRAMS)	SUGAR (TSPS)
Bottled, Carton, and Canned					
Carrot	8 fl oz	94	20	14	3½
Tomato Juice	8 fl oz	50	111	8	2
V-8 Juice	8 fl oz	50	11	8	2

Soft Drinks and Carbonated Beverages

Because there are so many different types, brand-name soft drinks are not included in this table. Virtually all soft drinks of the same type contain similar amounts of calories and sugar. Listed below you'll find the popular flavors, which you can compare to your favorite brand-name

FOOD	SERVING SIZE	CALORIES	CARBO-HYDRATES (GRAMS)	SUGAR (GRAMS)	SUGAR (TSPS)

products. Although most fast food restaurants carry brand-name soft drinks, they often do not include them in the total meal nutrient counts. You will find many of the brand-names listed in the Fast Foods section beginning on page 165.

FOOD	SERVING SIZE	CALORIES	CARBO-HYDRATES (GRAMS)	SUGAR (GRAMS)	SUGAR (TSPS)
Cola	12 fl oz	160	41	43	10¼
Cream soda	12 fl oz	189	49	49	12¼
Ginger ale	12 fl oz	125	32	32	8
Grape soda	12 fl oz	160	42	42	10½
Lemon-lime soda	12 fl oz	147	36	36	9
Orange soda	12 fl oz	180	46	46	11½
Quinine water	12 fl oz	130	43	43	8½
Root beer	12 fl oz	152	42	42	10½
Tonic water	12 fl oz	140	36	36	9

Tea

FOOD	SERVING SIZE	CALORIES	CARBO-HYDRATES (GRAMS)	SUGAR (GRAMS)	SUGAR (TSPS)
Botanica					
Frozen tea, all varieties	8 fl oz	208	50	30	7½
General Foods International Flavored Instant Tea, all varities	8 fl oz	70	13	10–11	2½–2¾
Nestea					
Plain, lemon	2 tbsp in 8 fl oz water	80	19	19	4½
Earl Grey	2 tbsp in 8 fl oz water	68	18	18	4½
Extra Sweet w/ Lemon	2 tbsp in 8 fl oz water	100	27	27	6¾

FOOD	SERVING SIZE	CALORIES	CARBO-HYDRATES (GRAMS)	SUGAR (GRAMS)	SUGAR (TSPS)

BREAKFAST CEREALS

Always remember to read the labels on cereal boxes, as manufacturers may sometimes change the name or formulation of a product if sales are low. Serving sizes listed on different cereal boxes range from one-third to one cup and are sometimes listed in ounces, so it is often difficult to compare the sugar content of one cereal to another without performing mind-bending calculations. Cereals that contain less than two teaspoons of sugar are not mentioned below. These cereals include rice puffs, corn puffs, wheat puffs, cornflakes, and many bran cereals. (Health Valley Cereals have between one and two teaspoons of sugar per serving.) Watch out for cereals that have more than 50 percent of their calories from sugar. These include Cinnamon Crunch, Lucky Charms, Cocoa Pebbles, Apple Jacks, Fruity Pebbles, King Vitamin, Sugar Smacks, and Super Orange Crisp.

Instant

FOOD	SERVING SIZE	CALORIES	CARBO-HYDRATES (GRAMS)	SUGAR (GRAMS)	SUGAR (TSPS)
Fantastic Foods					
All varieties	1 pkg	170–180	37–42	12–16	3–4
Health Valley					
Apple Cinnamon Flavor	1 pkg	210	41	9	2¼
Banana Nut Flavor	1 pkg	240	45	9	2¼
Maple Madness	1 pkg	240	47	19	4¾
Terrific 10 Grain	1 pkg	220	41	8	2
Nabisco					
Cream of Wheat, all flavored cereals	1 pkg	130	29	12–13	3–3¼
Quaker					
Instant Oatmeal					
Apples & Cinnamon	1 pkg	130	27	11	2¾

FOOD	SERVING SIZE	CALORIES	CARBO-HYDRATES (GRAMS)	SUGAR (GRAMS)	SUGAR (TSPS)
Quaker (continued)					
Instant Oatmeal Bananas & Cream	1 pkg	130	26	11	2¾
Instant Oatmeal Blueberries & Cream	1 pkg	130	26	11	2¾
Instant Oatmeal Cinnamon & Spice	1 pkg	170	36	16	4
Instant Oatmeal Maple & Brown Sugar	1 pkg	160	33	13	3¼
Instant Oatmeal Peaches & Cream	1 pkg	140	27	12	3
Instant Oatmeal Raisin & Spices	1 pkg	150	33	16	4
Instant Oatmeal Raisin, Date & Walnut	1 pkg	140	27	13	3¼
Instant Oatmeal Strawberries & Cream	1 pkg	140	27	11	2¾
Kid's Choice Instant Oatmeal, all flavors	1 pkg	154–159	29–32	11–15	2¾–3¾
Quick'n Hearty Oatmeal Microwave Apple Spice	1 pkg	170	35	15	3¾
Quick'n Hearty Oatmeal Microwave Brown Sugar Cinnamon	1 pkg	150	31	12	3
Quick'n Hearty Oatmeal Microwave Cinnamon Double Raisin	1 pkg	170	35	16	4
Quick'n Hearty Oatmeal Microwave Honey Bran	1 pkg	150	30	12	3
Ready to Eat					
Arrowhead Mills					
Maple Buckwheat Flakes	1 cup	160	35	9	2¼

FOOD	SERVING SIZE	CALORIES	CARBO-HYDRATES (GRAMS)	SUGAR (GRAMS)	SUGAR (TSPS)
Arrowhead Mills (continued)					
Raisin Bran	1 cup	190	41	10	2½
Rice Flakes	1 cup	80	19	9	2¼
Shredded Wheat, Sweetened	1 cup	200	44	12	3
Wild Ancient Wheat Flakes	1 cup	160	37	10	2½
Barbara's					
Apple Cinnamon Toasted O's	¾ cup	110	24	11	2¾
Bite Size Shredded Oats	1¼ cup	220	46	12	3
Cocoa Crunch Stars	1 cup	110	26	8	2
Frosted Corn Flakes	1 cup	110	27	8	2
Honey Crunch Stars	1 cup	110	26	8	2
Honey Nut Toasted O's	¾ cup	120	23	11	2¾
Organic Fruity Punch	1 cup	110	26	8	2
Organic Ultra Minis Frosted	¾ cup	190	46	12	3
Betty Crocker					
Dutch Apple	1 cup	220	47	18	4½
Streusel	¾ cup	120	25	9	2¼
Erewhon					
Raisin Bran	1 cup	170	28	10	2½
General Mills					
Basic 4	1 cup	200	43	14	3½
Boo Berry	1 cup	120	27	14	3½
Cheerios, Apple Cinnamon	1 cup	157	33	18	4½
Cheerios, Frosted	1 cup	115	26	14	3½
Cheerios, Honey Nut	1 cup	126	27	13	3¼
Cheerios Team	1 cup	120	25	11	2¾
Cinnamon Grahams	¾ cup	120	26	11	2¾
Cinnamon Toast Crunch	¾ cup	130	24	10	2½
Cocoa Puffs	1 cup	120	27	14	3½

FOOD	SERVING SIZE	CALORIES	CARBO-HYDRATES (GRAMS)	SUGAR (GRAMS)	SUGAR (TSPS)
General Mills (continued)					
Corn Flakes, Frosted	1 cup	161	37	14	3½
Count Chocula	1 cup	120	26	14	3½
Crispy Wheaties 'n Raisins	1 cup	190	44	20	5
Frankenberry	1 cup	120	27	14	3½
French Toast Crunch	1 cup	120	26	12	3
Golden Grahams	¾ cup	120	25	11	2¾
Granola, fruit, low fat	⅔ cup	210	44	19	4¾
Granola, low fat	1 cup	360	53	16	4
Honey Nut Clusters	1 cup	210	46	16	4
Kix Berry Berry	1 cup	160	35	12	3
Lucky Charms	1 cup	120	25	13	3¼
Multi-Bran Chex	1 cup	200	49	12	3
Nesquik Chocolate	¾ cup	120	25	12	3
Oatmeal Crisp	1 cup	220	42	16	4
Oatmeal Crisp Almond	1 cup	220	42	15	3¾
Oatmeal Crisp Apple	1 cup	210	46	19	4¾
Oatmeal Crisp Raisin	1 cup	210	44	19	4¾
Raisin Nut Bran	¾ cup	200	41	16	4
Reese's Peanut Butter Puffs	¾ cup	130	24	13	3¼
S'mores Grahams	¾ cup	120	26	13	3¼
Sun Crunchers	1 cup	220	45	16	4
Total Brown Sugar & Oats	¾ cup	110	25	9	2¼
Total Raisin Bran	1 cup	180	43	19	4¾
Trix	1 cup	120	26	13	3¼
Wheaties, Honey Frosted	¾ cup	110	27	12	3
Wheaties Raisin Bran	1 cup	180	45	18	4½

FOOD	SERVING SIZE	CALORIES	CARBO-HYDRATES (GRAMS)	SUGAR (GRAMS)	SUGAR (TSPS)
Grist Mill					
Apple Cinnamon Natural	½ cup	260	36	15	3¾
Bran	½ cup	250	37	8	2
Oat & Honey Natural	½ cup	270	34	11	2¾
Oat Honey & Raisin Natural	½ cup	260	35	14	3½
Health Valley					
Bran w/ Apples & Cinnamon	⅓ cup	160	41	10	2½
Bran w/ Raisins	⅓ cup	160	40	10	2½
Banana Gone Nuts Crunches & Flakes	¾ cup	200	41	11	2¾
Cranberry Crunch	¾ cup	190	38	10	2½
Golden Flax	½ cup	190	38	9	2¼
Honey Nut O's	¾ cup	120	24	8	2
Low Fat Granola, all flavors	⅔ cup	190	42	10	2½
Raspberry Rhapsody Cereal	¾ cup	200	41	10	2½
Real Oat Bran-Almond Crunch	½ cup	200	34	9	2¼
Healthy Choice					
Almond Crunch with Raisins	1 cup	210	45	15	3¾
Multi-grain Flakes	½ oz	142	35	9	2¼
Kellogg's					
All Bran	1 cup	164	47	12	3
Apple Cinnamon Squares	1 cup	242	59	16	4
Apple Jacks	1 cup	127	30	16	4
Apple Raisin Crunch	1 cup	178	45	15	3¾
Blueberry Squares	1 cup	238	57	15	3¾
Bran Buds	1 cup	251	73	24	6
Cinnamon Mini Buns	1 cup	154	36	16	4

FOOD	SERVING SIZE	CALORIES	CARBO-HYDRATES (GRAMS)	SUGAR (GRAMS)	SUGAR (TSPS)
Kellogg's (continued)					
Cocoa Krispies	1 cup	159	36	17	4¼
Common Sense	1 cup	145	31	8	2
Corn Pops	1 cup	118	28	13	3¼
Cracklin' Oat Bran	1 cup	266	47	21	5¼
Double Dip Crunch	1 cup	149	36	15	3¾
Fruit Loops	1 cup	125	28	15	3¾
Frosted Bran	1 cup	203	51	19	4¾
Frosted Flakes	1 cup	158	37	17	4¼
Frosted Mini Wheats	1 cup	173	42	18	4½
Fruity Marshmallow Crispies	1 cup	140	33	17	4¼
Honey Crunch Corn Flakes	1 cup	147	35	13	3¼
Honey Smacks Granola	¾ cup	120	30	10	2½
Just Right Fruit & Nut	1 cup	220	26	10	2½
Low Fat Granola	½ cup	190	39	14	3½
Low Fat Granola w/ Raisins	⅔ cup	220	48	17	4¼
Mini-Wheels, all flavors	¾ cup	180	44	12	3
Muselix, Apple & Almond Crunch	1 cup	272	53	12	3
Mueslix, Raisin & Almond Crunch w/ Dates	⅔ cup	200	41	17	4¼
Nut & Honey Crunch	⅔ cup	150	31	12	3
Raisin Bran	1 cup	200	47	18	4½
Raisin Squares	1 cup	241	55	15	3¾
Razzle Dazzle Rice Krispies	¾ cup	110	25	10	2½
Rice Krispies, Cinnamon & Apple	1 cup	145	35	15	3¾
Rice Krispies, Frosted	1 cup	132	32	13	3¼

FOOD	SERVING SIZE	CALORIES	CARBO-HYDRATES (GRAMS)	SUGAR (GRAMS)	SUGAR (TSPS)
Kellogg's (continued)					
Rice Krispies Treats	¾ cup	120	26	9	2¼
Strawberry Squares	1 cup	228	53	12	3
Temptations, French Vanilla Almond	1 cup	139	29	10	2½
Temptations, Honey Roasted Pecan	1 cup	175	35	14	3½
Kolin					
Crispy Oats	1 cup	190	40	9	2¼
Oat Muesli Fruit	¾ cup	200	39	12	3
Kraft					
Morning Traditions Banana Nut Crunch	1 cup	250	43	12	3
Morning Traditions Blueberry Morning	1¼ cup	220	43	13	3¼
Morning Traditions Cranberry Almond Crunch	1 cup	220	44	15	3¾
Morning Traditions Great Grains, Raisins, Dates & Pecans	⅔ cup	210	39	14	3½
Morning Traditions					
Banana Nut Crunch	1 cup	250	43	12	3
Blueberry Morning	1¼ cup	220	43	13	3¼
Cranberry Almond Crunch	1 cup	220	44	15	3¾
Great Grains, Crunchy Pecan	⅔ cup	220	38	9	2¼
Great Grains, Raisins, Dates & Pecans	⅔ cup	210	39	14	3½
Nabisco					
100% Bran Flakes	1 cup	178	48	16	4
Frosted Shredded Wheat Bite Size	1 cup	190	44	12	3

FOOD	SERVING SIZE	CALORIES	CARBO-HYDRATES (GRAMS)	SUGAR (GRAMS)	SUGAR (TSPS)
Nabisco (continued)					
Fruit Wheats, all varieties	1 cup	221–227	53–55	13–16	3¼–4
Honey Nut Shredded Wheat Bite Size	1 cup	200	43	12	3
Team Flakes	1 cup	178	40	8	2
Post					
Alpha-Bits	1 cup	130	27	13	3¼
Blueberry Morning	1 cup	186	36	11	2¾
Banana Nut Crunch	1 cup	250	43	11	2¾
Bran'nola Original	1 cup	400	86	30	7½
Bran'nola w/ Raisins	1 cup	400	88	39	9¾
Cocoa Pebbles	¾ cup	120	26	13	3¼
C.W. Post	1 cup	421	72	22	5½
C. W. Post w/ Raisins	1 cup	446	74	25	6¼
Fruit & Fibre, all varieties	1 cup	193–221	43–46	15–18	3¾–4½
Fruity PEBBLES	¾ cup	110	24	12	3
Granola, Hearty	1 cup	422	68	23	5¾
Great Grains, Raisin, Dates & Pecans	1 cup	319	59	20	5
Honey Bunches of Oats w/ and w/o Almonds	1 cup	172	32	8	2
Honeycomb	1⅓ cup	110	26	11	2¾
Oat Flakes	1 cup	180	36	11	2¾
Raisin Bran	1 cup	190	47	20	5
Super Golden Crisp	1 cup	123	30	17	4¼
Quaker					
Cap'n Crunch Crunchberries	¾ cup	113	24	12	3
Cap'n Crunch Original	¾ cup	107	23	12	3

FOOD	SERVING SIZE	CALORIES	CARBO-HYDRATES (GRAMS)	SUGAR (GRAMS)	SUGAR (TSPS)
Quaker (continued)					
Cap'n Crunch Peanut Butter Crunch	¾ cup	119	22	9	2¼
Cinnamon Oatmeal Squares	1 cup	232	42	10	2½
Cocoa Blasts	1 cup	129	29	16	4
Corn Quakes	¾ cup	121	25	11	2¾
Corn Bran	1 cup	120	30	8	2
Frosted Flakes	¾ cup	116	27	12	3
Fruitany Ohs	1 cup	121	27	13	3¼
Granola Oats & Honey	1 cup	462	71	25	6¼
Granola Natural w/ Raisins	1 cup	437	72	25	6¼
Granola Natural w/ Raisins & Dates	1 cup	496	72	19	4¾
Honey Graham Oh!s	¾ cup	112	22	11	2¾
Honey Nut Toasted Oatmeal	1 cup	191	39	13	3¼
Life Oat Cinnamon	¾ cup	120	26	10	2½
Marshmallow Safari	¾ cup	119	25	14	3½
Oatmeal Squares, Almond	1 cup	216	43	9	2¼
Quisp/Sweet Crunch	1 cup	121	26	12	3
Sweet Puffs	1 cup	133	30	17	4¼
Ralston Purina					
Almond Delight	1 cup	210	41	12	3
Bran Chex	1 cup	156	39	9	2¼
Cocoa Crispy Rice	1 cup	200	45	18	4½
Cocoa Crunchies	¾ cup	120	26	13	3¼
Cookie Crisp	1 cup	120	25	12	3
Crisp Crunch	¾ cup	120	26	14	3½
Frosted Flakes	¾ cup	120	28	11	2¾

FOOD	SERVING SIZE	CALORIES	CARBO-HYDRATES (GRAMS)	SUGAR (GRAMS)	SUGAR (TSPS)
Ralston Purina (continued)					
Fruit Rings	¾ cup	120	23	12	3
Magic Stair	¾ cup	120	26	11	2¾
Muesli Blueberry Pecan	1 cup	200	41	14	3½
Muesli Cranberry Walnut	¾ cup	200	40	14	3½
Muesli Peach Pecan	¾ cup	200	39	12	3
Muesli Raspberry Almond	¾ cup	220	44	14	3½
Muesli Strawberry Pecan	1 cup	210	41	14	3½
Raisin Bran	¾ cup	190	41	16	4
Tasteeos Apple Cinnamon	1 cup	130	27	10	2½
Tasteeos Honey Nut	1 cup	130	28	10	2½
Sunbelt					
Granola Banana Nut	1.9 oz	254	34	12	3
Granola Fruit & Nut	1.9 oz	246	39	16	4
Granola Low Fat	1.9 oz	220	44	20	5
Muesli	1.9 oz	210	44	17	4¼
Uncle Roy's					
Muesli	1 cup	340	64	16	4

CANDY

Most of the calories in candy, if not all of them, come from sugar. There are approximately 15 to 20 calories of sugar per teaspoon, so if your candy contains 11¼ teaspoons of sugar, there are approximately 168 to 225 calories from sugar in that product. That's quite a bit! Also beware that hydrogenated fat, which was discussed on page 26, is often the second or third ingredient in candy.

When the serving size of a candy is listed below in ounces or

FOOD	SERVING SIZE	CALORIES	CARBO-HYDRATES (GRAMS)	SUGAR (GRAMS)	SUGAR (TSPS)

grams, it is usually a single piece. Sometimes, manufactures may change the serving size, so read your labels. Also, many candies come in different sizes, including fun size, trick or treat size, munch size, junior size, kid size, king size, mini size, small size, snack size, super size, regular size, and others! This, of course, makes it difficult for the consumer to compare the nutritional facts of one product with another.

FOOD	SERVING SIZE	CALORIES	CARBO-HYDRATES (GRAMS)	SUGAR (GRAMS)	SUGAR (TSPS)
Generic					
Candy Corn	¼ cup	182	45	45	11¼
Caramels, plain or chocolate	1 oz	115	26	22	5½
Chocolate, milk	1.5 oz	260	26	24	6
Chocolate, milk w/ almonds	1.5 oz	216	21	18	4½
Chocolate, milk w/ rice cereal	1 oz	140	18	18	4½
Chocolate, milk w/ peanuts	10 oz	208	19	15	3¾
Fondant, uncoated (mints, and others)	1 oz	105	27	27	6¾
Fudge, chocolate, plain	1 oz	115	21	21	5¼
Gum drops	1 oz	100	25	25	6¼
Hard candy	1 oz	110	28	28	7
Jelly beans	10	40	11	11	2¾
Licorice	1 oz	103	26	26	6¼
Marshmallows, large	4	90	35	23	5¾
Marshmallows, mini size	1 cup	146	37	26	6½
Abba Zabba					
Bar	2 oz	250	48	23	5¾
Andes					
Chocolate Covered Mint Patty	1 patty	60	13	12	3
Creme de Menthe Chocolate Thins	8 pieces	210	22	21	5¼

FOOD	SERVING SIZE	CALORIES	CARBO-HYDRATES (GRAMS)	SUGAR (GRAMS)	SUGAR (TSPS)
Bit-O-Honey					
Pieces	1.7 oz	186	39	23	4¾
Bonus Bar					
Bar	2.1 oz	290	34	17	4¼
Brach's					
Candy Corn	1 oz	100	26	26	6½
High C Orange Slices	3 slices	150	38	30	7½
Star Brites Peppermints	1 oz	120	36	28	7
Wild & Fruity Gummy Worms	5 pieces	150	35	25	6¼
Brock					
Butterscotch Discs	3 pieces	70	17	11	2¾
Candy Corn	21 pieces	150	37	29	7¼
Candy Rolls	2 pieces	50	12	12	3
Caramel Dots	3 pieces	140	25	14	3½
Cinnamon Discs	3 pieces	70	17	11	2¾
Circus Peanuts	11 pieces	260	65	60	15
Coconut Mountains	4 pieces	170	29	24	6
Fruit Basket	3 pieces	60	15	13	3¼
Fruit Kisses	3 pieces	70	17	11	2¾
Glitters	2 pieces	50	13	8	2
Gummy Bears	5 pieces	130	30	25	6¼
Gummy Squirms	5 pieces	120	28	24	6
Jelly Beans	12 pieces	140	36	26	6½
Lemon Drops	3 pieces	60	14	9	2¼
Orange Slices	4 pieces	140	36	27	6¾
Party Mints	9 pieces	60	15	15	3¾
Peanut Butter Crunch	3 pieces	80	15	10	2½

FOOD	SERVING SIZE	CALORIES	CARBO-HYDRATES (GRAMS)	SUGAR (GRAMS)	SUGAR (TSPS)
Brock (continued)					
Pops Assorted	2 pieces	60	15	10	2½
Sour Balls	3 pieces	70	17	11	2¾
Sour Sharks	23 pieces	30	60	45	11¼
Spearmint Starlights	3 pieces	60	16	10	2½
Spice Drops	12 pieces	130	33	24	6
Starlight Mints	3 pieces	60	16	10	2½
Toffee	6 pieces	170	31	27	6¾
Brown & Haley					
Almond Roca	3 pieces	210	17	17	4¼
Cadbury's					
Almond	9 blocks of 5 oz bar	280	41	40	10
Caramello	5 blocks of 5 oz bar	190	25	19	4¾
Dairy Milk Bar	5 blocks of 5 oz bar	220	24	21	5¼
Charm's					
All varieties	1 piece	70	17–18	14–17	3½–4¼
Cracker Jack's					
Popcorn	1 pkg	150	30	19	4¾
Crunch Fun Size	4 pkg	140	34	24	6
Dove					
Chocolate Miniatures	7 pieces	220	26	21	5¼
Dark Chocolate	1.5 oz	230	26	22	5½
Milk Chocolate	1.3 oz	200	22	21	5¼
Milk Chocolate	1.5 oz	230	25	24	6
Milk Chocolate Miniatures	7 pieces	230	25	24	6
Dream					
Caramel & Nougat in Milk Chocolate	1 piece	90	21	8	2

FOOD	SERVING SIZE	CALORIES	CARBO-HYDRATES (GRAMS)	SUGAR (GRAMS)	SUGAR (TSPS)
Dum Dums					
Pieces	1 oz	100	26	26	6½
Estee					
Dark Chocolate	1.4 oz	200	23	15	3¾
Gum Drops Assorted Fruit	23 pieces	140	36	30	7½
Milk Chocolate	1.4 oz	230	17	15	3¾
Milk Chocolate w/ Almonds	1.4 oz	230	16	14	3½
Milk Chocolate w/ Crisp Rice	1.4 oz	370	29	24	6
Milk Chocolate w/ Fruit & Nuts	1.4 oz	220	18	15	3¾
Mint Chocolate	1.4 oz	200	23	15	3¾
Peanut Butter Cups	1.3 oz	200	19	13	3¼
Favorite Brand					
Candy Corn	24 pieces	150	37	34	8½
Cinnamon Imperials	52 pieces	80	14	12	3
Circus Peanuts	5 pieces	160	39	33	8¼
Gummallo Apple Ring	5 pieces	120	27	20	5
Gummallo Peach Ring	5 pieces	120	27	20	5
Gummi Bears	18 pieces	130	30	19	4¾
Gummi Dinos	7 pieces	120	28	18	4½
Gummi Worms	4 pieces	130	29	18	4½
Marshmallow Eggs	3 pieces	140	34	32	8
Neon Worms	4 pieces	120	28	22	5½
Sour Gummi Bears	16 pieces	110	26	20	5
Sour Gummi Worms	4 pieces	130	29	23	5¾
Ferro Rocher					
Hazelnut Chocolate	2 pieces	150	11	11	2¾

FOOD	SERVING SIZE	CALORIES	CARBO-HYDRATES (GRAMS)	SUGAR (GRAMS)	SUGAR (TSPS)
Ghirardelli					
Cookies & Cream	½ of 3 oz bar	380	37	33	8¼
Dark Chocolate	½ of 3 oz bar	210	26	21	5¼
Milk Chocolate w/ & w/o almonds	½ of 3 oz bar	220	25	23	5¾
Mint Squares	4 pieces	220	26	24	6
Raspberries & Cream	½ of 3 oz bar	230	25	25	6¼
Godiva					
Almond Butter Dome	3 pieces	240	19	14	3½
Bouchee Au Chocolate	1 piece	210	25	18	4½
Bouchee Ivory Raspberry	1 piece	160	17	11	2¾
Gold Ballotin	3 pieces	210	27	21	5¼
Truffle Amaretto Di Saranno	2 pieces	210	24	17	4¼
Truffle Deluxe Liqueur	2 pieces	210	23	16	4
Goldberg's					
Peanut Chews	3 pieces	180	22	14	3½
Goobers					
Peanuts	1 pkg	210	19	16	4
Good and Plenty					
Snack Size	3 boxes	140	34	24	6
Haviland					
Chocolate Covered Thin Mints	6 pieces	170	33	32	8
Heath					
Bar	1.6 oz	210	25	24	6
Hershey's					
Almond Joy	1.7 oz	240	29	22	5½
Cookies 'n Cream and Cookies and Mint	1.6 oz	227	24	20	5
Crackel Bar	1 bar	218	25	21	5¼

FOOD	SERVING SIZE	CALORIES	CARBO-HYDRATES (GRAMS)	SUGAR (GRAMS)	SUGAR (TSPS)
Hershey's (continued)					
5th Ave.	2 oz	197	26	18	4½
Hugs	8 pieces	210	23	20	5
Hugs w/ Almonds	9 pieces	230	21	19	4¾
Kisses	9 pieces	230	24	21	5¼
Kisses w/ Almonds	9 pieces	230	21	19	4¾
KitKat	1.5 oz	220	27	22	5½
Milk Chocolate	1.5 oz	233	25	22	5½
Milk Chocolate w/ Almonds	1.4 oz	230	20	18	4½
Milk Duds	13 pieces	170	28	19	4¾
Mini Kisses	11 pieces	82	9	8	2
Mr. Goodbar	1.7 oz	270	25	22	5½
Nuggets	4 pieces	210	20	16	4
Pay Day	1.8 oz	240	28	20	5
Reese's Peanut Butter Cups	1.8 oz	280	26	22	5½
Reese's Pieces	1 bag	260	32	27	6¾
Reese's Sticks	1 pkg	120	11	8	2
Rolo Caramels	9 pieces	219	28	26	6½
Skor English Toffee Bar	1.4 oz	220	23	21	5¼
Solitaires	2.8 oz	445	37	29	7¼
Sweet Escape, all varieties	1.1 oz	70–80	14–20	11–19	2¾–4¾
Symphony Milk Chocolate	4 blocks of 7 oz bar	220	22	20	5
Symphony Milk Chocolate w/ Almonds & Toffee Chips	4 blocks of 7 oz bar	220	20	17	4¼
Tastetations	3 pieces	60	12	10	2½
Whatchamacallit	1.7 oz	220	29	21	5¼

FOOD	SERVING SIZE	CALORIES	CARBO-HYDRATES (GRAMS)	SUGAR (GRAMS)	SUGAR (TSPS)
Hershey's (continued)					
Whoppers Malted Milk Balls	18 pieces	180	29	29	7¼
Jolly Rancher					
All varieties	3 pieces	60	14	9	2¼
Joyva					
Halvah Chocolate Covered	2 oz	380	20	19	4¾
Jells Raspberry	3 pieces	200	25	24	6
Joys Raspberry	1 piece	200	25	24	6
Marshmallow Twists Chocolate Covered	1.5 oz	190	23	21	5¼
Rings Orange & Raspberry	3 pieces	190	23	22	5½
Sticks Orange	3 pieces	200	25	24	6
Twists Vanilla & Cherry	2 pieces	190	21	23	5¾
Junior Mints					
Pieces	1 pkg	75	16	16	4
Kraft					
Butter Mints and Party Mints	7 pieces	60	14	14	3½
Caramels	5 pieces	170	32	27	6¾
Peanut Brittle	5 pieces	170	29	21	5¼
Laffy Taffy					
Chews	1 oz	110	25	25	6¼
Lifesavers					
Big Tablet Candy Cane	4 pieces	60	16	13	3¼
Cards 'N Candy	4 pieces	40	10	10	2½
Christmas Tin	4 pieces	60	16	13	3¼
Egg-Sortment	1 roll	40	10	10	2½
Fruit Juicers Lollipops	1 piece	40	10	10	2½
Gummi Bunnies	3 pkg	40	34	23	5¾

FOOD	SERVING SIZE	CALORIES	CARBO-HYDRATES (GRAMS)	SUGAR (GRAMS)	SUGAR (TSPS)
Lifesavers (continued)					
Gummi Savers, all flavors	10 pieces	120	30	23	5¾
Gummi Savers, Crystal Craze	12 pieces	130	31	23	5¾
Lollipops, all flavors	1 piece	40	10–11	7–11	1¾-2¾
Peppomint	4 pieces	60	15	15	¾
Sack'it, all flavors	4 pieces	60	16	13–15	3¼–3¾
LIndt					
Bittersweet	2.5 oz	220	21	18	4½
Lindor Truffles	2.5 oz	230	16	16	4
Milk Chocolate	2.5 oz	210	23	21	5¼
Milk Chocolate w/ Almonds	2.5 oz	240	20	19	4¾
Milk Chocolate w/ Cherries	2.5 oz	190	25	24	6
Milk Chocolate w/ Hazelnuts	2.5 oz	230	19	18	4½
Milk Chocolate w/ Pistachios	2.5 oz	250	20	20	5
Milk Chocolate w/ Raspberries	2.5 oz	200	25	25	6¼
White Chocolate	2.5 oz	240	17	17	4¼
M & M's-Mars					
Mars Almond Bar, fun size	2 pkg	190	23	20	5
Mars Almond Bar	1.8 oz	240	31	26	6½
Milky Way dark and light	1.8 oz	220	36	30	7½
Milky Way dark and light, fun size	2 pkg	180	28	24	6
M & M's Almond	1.5 oz	220	24	21	5¼
M & M's Mint	1.5 oz	200	30	27	6¾
M & M's Peanut, fun size	1 pkg	110	13	11	2¾
M & M's Peanut	1.7 oz	253	30	25	6¼

FOOD	SERVING SIZE	CALORIES	CARBO-HYDRATES (GRAMS)	SUGAR (GRAMS)	SUGAR (TSPS)
M & M's-Mars (continued)					
M & M's Peanut Butter, fun size	1 pkg	110	12	10	2½
M & M's Peanut Butter	1.5 oz	220	25	20	5
M & M's Plain, fun size	1 pkg	100	15	13	3¼
M & M's Plain	1.7 oz	230	34	21	5¼
Snickers	2.1 oz	280	36	30	7½
Snickers, fun size	2 pieces	190	24	20	5
Snickers Miniatures	4 pieces	170	22	18	4½
Snickers Peanut Butter	2 oz	310	28	23	5¾
3 Musketeers	2.1 oz	260	46	40	10
Twix Caramel	2 oz	284	37	27	6¾
Twix Peanut Butter	1.9 oz	286	29	19	4¾
Milkshake					
Bar	1.8 oz	220	38	25	6¼
Mounds					
Bar	1.9 oz	260	31	21	5¼
Mr. Goodbar					
Bar	1.7 oz	290	23	21	5¼
Necco					
Thin Mints	6 pieces	170	33	32	8
Wafers	1 oz	110	27	27	6¾
Nestlé					
Baby Ruth	2.1 oz	270	36	27	6¾
Baby Ruth, fun size	1.4 oz	130	17	13	4¼
Buncha Crunch	1.4 oz	90	26	20	5
Butterfinger	2.1 oz	270	42	29	7¼
Chocolate cream	3 pieces	190	21	19	4¾
Chunky Bar	1.4 oz	210	24	21	5¼

FOOD	SERVING SIZE	CALORIES	CARBO-HYDRATES (GRAMS)	SUGAR (GRAMS)	SUGAR (TSPS)
Nestlé (continued)					
Crunch	1.5 oz	230	29	24	6
Crunch, fun size	4 bars	210	26	22	5½
Flipz, Milk Chocolate	1 oz	130	20	10	2½
Flipz, Peanut Butter	1 oz	140	19	8	2
Flipz, White Fudge	1 oz	130	19	11	2¾
Milk Chocolate, regular size	2.5 oz	370	40	37	9¼
Mocha Crunch	1 oz	200	21	18	4½
Oh Henry !	1 oz	120	16	12	3
100 Grand	1 oz	200	30	27	6¾
Raisinets	1 bag	190	31	27	6¾
Sno Caps	1 box	300	48	38	9½
Toasted Coconut	4 pieces	240	26	25	6¼
Treasure, Caramel	3 pieces	180	22	19	4¾
Treasure, Peanut Butter	4 pieces	250	23	21	5¼
Turtles	2 pieces	160	20	13	3¼
White Crunch	1 piece	110	23	20	5
Newman's Own					
Butter Toffee Crunch	½ bar	220	24	22	5½
Espresso Sweet Dark Chocolate	1 piece	190	19	15	3¾
Pearson's					
Mint Patties	5 pieces	150	31	27	6¾
Nut Roll	1 piece	350	40	29	7¼
Planters					
Original Peanut Bar	1 pkg	230	22	13	3¼
Riesen					
Chocolate Chews	5 pieces	180	29	20	5

FOOD	SERVING SIZE	CALORIES	CARBO-HYDRATES (GRAMS)	SUGAR (GRAMS)	SUGAR (TSPS)
Russell Stover					
Assorted Chocolates	3 pieces	180	29	25	5½
Pecan Rolls	2 oz	300	26	21	4¼
Truffle Golf Balls	1 piece	200	22	21	5¼
Skittles					
Original	1.5 oz	170	38	32	8
Original, fun size	2 pkg	180	41	35	8¾
Tropical	1.5 oz	170	38	32	8
Wild Berry	1.5 oz	170	38	32	8
Wild Berry, fun size	2 pkg	160	36	30	7½
Toblerone					
Swiss Chocolate in Honey & Almond Nougat	1.2 oz	180	21	20	5
Tootsie					
Midges	6 pieces	160	33	30	7½
Tootsie Roll	½ bar	130	27	24	6
Twizzlers					
Candy	1.4 oz	130	30	14	3½
Cherry Bits Licorice	3.8 oz	135	31	17	4¼
Pull-N-Peel Cherry	1.1 oz	110	23	13	3¼
Strawberry Bits Licorice	2.5 oz	237	54	26	6½
Whitman's					
Little Ambassadors	7 pieces	190	26	22	5½
Pecan Delight	2 oz	310	27	17	4¼
Pecan Roll	2 oz	300	26	21	5¼
Sampler, assorted and dark chocolate	3 pieces	190–200	25–27	19–22	4¾–5½
Snoopy Treats, snack size	1 pkg	80	24	18	4½

FOOD	SERVING SIZE	CALORIES	CARBO-HYDRATES (GRAMS)	SUGAR (GRAMS)	SUGAR (TSPS)
York					
Peppermint Pattie, snack size	1 snack size	57	11	8	2
Peppermint Pattie	1.5 oz	180	34	27	6¾
Zero					
Bar	2 oz	170	28	21	5¼

DAIRY

Dairy products naturally contain sugar in the form of lactose and galactose. When fruit is added to a dairy product, it increases the sugar content of that particular food. Quite often, there is no way to tell how much extra sugar has been added to flavored dairy products. Cream, whipped cream, and half and half, which are not listed in this section, contain about ½ teaspoon of natural sugar for every 2 tablespoons.

Cottage Cheese

FOOD	SERVING SIZE	CALORIES	CARBO-HYDRATES (GRAMS)	SUGAR (GRAMS)	SUGAR (TSPS)
Friendship					
4% Milk fat w/ Pineapple	½ cup	140	14	14	2½
Low Fat w/ Pineapple	½ cup	120	16	15	2¾
Nonfat w/ Peach	½ cup	110	15	14	2½
Nonfat w/ Pineapple	½ cup	110	16	15	2¾
Knudsen					
Low Fat w/ Pineapple	½ cup	120	14	12	3
On the Go, Low Fat, all fruit flavors	½ cup	110	13	11–12	2¾–3
Peach & Pineapple	½ cup	110	15	14	3½

FOOD	SERVING SIZE	CALORIES	CARBO-HYDRATES (GRAMS)	SUGAR (GRAMS)	SUGAR (TSPS)

Ice Cream

There are many manufacturers of ice cream, and each offers a wide variety of choices—from the traditional plain vanilla to flavors like toasted walnut fudge, and from regular to low fat to nonfat. Breyers, for instance, has over 158 flavors! Quite often, the same combination of flavors will go by a different name depending on who produces it, making nutritional comparisons somewhat difficult. Also, the serving size tends to vary from product to product. Some brand-name ice creams have many more calories and much more sugar than others. (Compare, for instance, Ben & Jerry's to Friendly's.) Also, when the list of ingredients is long and the name of the product is tricky, chances are that there is more sugar in that product. So, buyer beware! And, if you like to eat your ice cream on a cone, keep in mind that some cones also contain sugar. There are three varieties of cones: cake cups with no sugar, sugar cones, and wafer cones. The sugar content of sugar cones and wafer cones ranges from ½ teaspoon to 4 teaspoons. Store brands seem to contain the least amount of sugar. Once again, read labels.

FOOD	SERVING SIZE	CALORIES	CARBO-HYDRATES (GRAMS)	SUGAR (GRAMS)	SUGAR (TSPS)
Generic					
Chocolate	½ cup	143	19	14	3½
Coffee	½ cup	150	15	14	3½
Strawberry	½ cup	127	18	15	3¾
Vanilla	½ cup	132	16	14	3½
Vanilla light	½ cup	130	18	16	4
Ben & Jerry's					
Cherry Garcia	½ cup	260	26	23	5¾
Chocolate Chip Cookie Dough	½ cup	280	28	25	6¼
Chocolate Fudge Brownie	½ cup	280	32	27	6¾

FOOD	SERVING SIZE	CALORIES	CARBO-HYDRATES (GRAMS)	SUGAR (GRAMS)	SUGAR (TSPS)
Ben & Jerry's (continued)					
Chunky Monkey	½ cup	310	31	24	6
Coffee Heath Bar Crunch	½ cup	290	29	27	6¾
Everything but the . . .	½ cup	370	30	27	6¾
From Russia w/ Buzz	½ cup	270	26	23	5¾
Half Baked	½ cup	280	33	30	7½
Jerry's Jubilee	½ cup	260	29	25	6¼
Mint Chocolate Cookie	½ cup	280	28	25	6¼
Monkey Bread	½ cup	310	29	26	6½
New York Super Fudge Chunk	½ cup	320	28	22	5½
Nutty Waffle Cone	½ cup	310	32	26	6½
Orange & Creme	½ cup	230	23	21	5¼
Phish Food	½ cup	290	38	27	6¾
Pulp Addiction	½ cup	240	25	22	5½
Southern Pecan Pie	½ cup	300	26	22	5½
Triple Caramel Chunk	½ cup	300	23	21	5¼
Urban Jumbo	½ cup	330	28	24	6
Vanilla Caramel Fudge	½ cup	290	33	28	7
Vanilla Heath Bar Crunch	½ cup	310	30	27	6¾
Breyers					
All varieties	½ cup	130–180	14–24	13–17	3¼–4¼
Friendly's					
All varieties	½ cup	150–200	14–24	11–19	2¾–4¾
Godiva					
All varieties	½ cup	280–340	26–32	23–28	5¾–7
Haagen-Dazs					
All varieties, except low fat	½ cup	240–370	21–29	19–28	4¾–7
Low fat, all varieties	½ cup	150–170	29–32	15–22	4¼–5½

FOOD	SERVING SIZE	CALORIES	CARBO-HYDRATES (GRAMS)	SUGAR (GRAMS)	SUGAR (TSPS)
Weight Watchers					
Chocolate Tornado	½ cup	149	26	22	5½
Cookie Dough Craze, light	½ cup	140	24	21	5¼
Praline Crunch, light	½ cup	140	25	21	5¼
Rocky Road, light	½ cup	140	23	17	4¼
Vanilla, light	½ cup	120	20	16	4

Ice Cream Bars

FOOD	SERVING SIZE	CALORIES	CARBO-HYDRATES (GRAMS)	SUGAR (GRAMS)	SUGAR (TSPS)
Ben & Jerry's					
Pop Chocolate Chip Cookie Dough	1 bar	450	48	38	9½
Pop English Toffee Crunch	1 bar	340	35	34	8½
Pop Vanilla	1 bar	360	30	70	17½
Dovebar					
Drumstick	1 bar	340–370	37–41	20–25	5–6¼
Good Humor Bar					
Reese's Peanut Butter Cup Bar	1 bar	250	24	21	5¼
All other varieties	1 bar	150	19	11–16	2¾–4
Haagen Dazs					
Bars, Single	1 bar	340–380	25–34	24–33	6–8½
Bars, Multi-pack	1 bar	280–320	20–28	19–27	4¾–7¾

Ice Cream Sandwiches

FOOD	SERVING SIZE	CALORIES	CARBO-HYDRATES (GRAMS)	SUGAR (GRAMS)	SUGAR (TSPS)
Klondike					
All varieties	1 sandwich	200–290	30–31	16–25	4–6¼
Nestlé					
All varieties	1 sandwich	180	27	12	2
Weight Watchers					
Vanilla	2.4 oz	160	30	14	3⅓

FOOD	SERVING SIZE	CALORIES	CARBO-HYDRATES (GRAMS)	SUGAR (GRAMS)	SUGAR (TSPS)
Ice Milk					
Soft serve chocolate w/ sugar cone	½ cup	70	11	10	4½
Soft serve vanilla w/ cake cone	½ cup	70	11	10	2½
Kefer					
French vanilla	8 oz	240	41	38	9½
Raspberry	8 oz	240	41	38	9½
Strawberry	8 oz	260	45	39	9¾
Milk					
Fresh					
Buttermilk, cultured	8 fl oz	99	12	12	3
Milk	8 fl oz	150	12	12	3
Milk, low fat	8 fl oz	104	12	12	3
Milk, nonfat	8 fl oz	86	12	11	2¾
Milk, Chocolate, low fat	8 fl oz	180	26	22	5½
Darigold					
Eggnog	8 fl oz	360	44	32	8
Eggnog, low fat	8 fl oz	240	44	38	9½
Canned or Dried					
Carnation					
Condensed, Sweetened	2 tbsp	130	22	22	5½
Evaporated Milk	½ cup	160	12	12	3
Evaporated Low-Fat Milk	2 tbsp	100	12	12	3
Evaporated Fat-Free Milk	2 tsbp	100	16	16	4
Nonfat Dry Milk	⅓ cup	80	12	12	3

FOOD	SERVING SIZE	CALORIES	CARBO-HYDRATES (GRAMS)	SUGAR (GRAMS)	SUGAR (TSPS)
Non Dairy Milk					
Goat's Milk	8 fl oz	168	11	11	2¾

Milk Shakes

FOOD	SERVING SIZE	CALORIES	CARBO-HYDRATES (GRAMS)	SUGAR (GRAMS)	SUGAR (TSPS)
D'Frosta					
Fruit, No Fat, Lactose Free, Black Raspberry	6 fl oz	150	37	29	7¼
Hood					
All varieties	8 fl oz	240	36–38	33–35	8¼–8¾
Parmalat					
Shake A Shake Chocolate	1 box (5 oz)	180	29	27	6¾
Shake A Shake Orange Vanilla	1 box (5 oz)	110	14	14	3½
Shake A Shake Vanilla	1 box (5 oz)	170	28	27	6¾

Milk Substitutes

The milk substitutes listed here have a high sugar content, but there are other milk substitutes that have very little sugar in them. Health Valley is one of the manufactures of low-sugar milk substitutes.

FOOD	SERVING SIZE	CALORIES	CARBO-HYDRATES (GRAMS)	SUGAR (GRAMS)	SUGAR (TSPS)
Eden Blend					
Original Blend	8 fl oz	120	16	12	3
Edensoy					
All varieties	8 fl oz	150	23	14–15	3½–3¾
Rice Dream					
Original	8 fl oz	120	25	11	2¾
Vitasoy					
Carob Supreme	8 fl oz	210	32	21	5¼
Cocoa Light	8 fl oz	130	25	17	4¼
Original Creamy	8 fl oz	160	14	9	2¼
Original Light	8 fl oz	90	15	9	2¼
Rich Cocoa	8 fl oz	220	32	19	4¾

FOOD	SERVING SIZE	CALORIES	CARBO-HYDRATES (GRAMS)	SUGAR (GRAMS)	SUGAR (TSPS)
Vitasoy (continued)					
Vanilla Light	8 fl oz	110	20	15	3¾
Vanilla Delite	8 fl oz	190	27	21	5¼

Sherbert

Sherbert usually contains some milk or cream, in addition to fruit (usually from concentrate) and many forms of sweetener, such as sugar, corn syrup, and high fructose corn syrup. In general, calories, carbohydrates, and sugar vary little from manufacturer to manufacturer.

FOOD	SERVING SIZE	CALORIES	CARBO-HYDRATES (GRAMS)	SUGAR (GRAMS)	SUGAR (TSPS)
Breyers					
All varieties	½ cup	110–120	26–28	19–21	4¾–5¼
Hood					
All varieties	½ cup	120	26	26	6½
Sealtest					
All varieties	½ cup	130	28	21	5¼

Sorbet

Sorbet usually does not contain milk or cream but is included here because it is often thought of as a dairy product, like ice cream or sherbert. The main ingredients in Dreyer's Boysenberry Sorbet are water, corn syrup, sugar, boysenberries, high fructose corn syrup, and boysenberry juice from concentrate. There are many different simple sugars in this dessert. The sugar content in sorbet is comparable to that in ice cream, but sorbet is lower in fat.

FOOD	SERVING SIZE	CALORIES	CARBO-HYDRATES (GRAMS)	SUGAR (GRAMS)	SUGAR (TSPS)
Dreyer's					
All varieties	½ cup	120–150	31–40	23–32	5¾-8
Haagen-Dazs					
All varieties	½ cup	120–130	28–33	20–29	5–7¼
Sorbet Bars	1	80–120	15–20	14–15	3½–3¾

FOOD	SERVING SIZE	CALORIES	CARBO-HYDRATES (GRAMS)	SUGAR (GRAMS)	SUGAR (TSPS)

Yogurt

Yogurt contains the natural sugars galactose and lactose. When fruit is added, it also contains natural fruit sugars. Usually, additional sugar is added. Plain yogurt without added sugar can have between 2½ to 4 grams of sugar per serving, depending on the fat content (often the lower the fat, the higher the sugar). Use this to calculate how much added sugar is in the fruit-flavored yogurt of your choice.

FOOD	SERVING SIZE	CALORIES	CARBO-HYDRATES (GRAMS)	SUGAR (GRAMS)	SUGAR (TSPS)
Breyers					
Low fat, all varieties	8 oz	220–240	38–44	38–44	9½–11
Breyers Light, all varieties	8 oz	120–130	21–23	17–19	4¼–4½
Breyers Smooth & Creamy, all varieties	8 oz	230–240	45–48	39–41	9¾–10¼
Colombo					
Banana Strawberry	8 oz	220	47	42	10½
Blackberry Burst	8 oz	220	47	42	10½
Other fruit flavors	8 oz	200	42	35	8¾
Other varieties	8 oz	160	32	26	6½
Plain, full fat (no sugar added)	8 oz	100	16	10	2½
Continental					
Fruit at Bottom, all flavors	8 oz	200	38	24	6
Dannon					
Danimals, all varieties	3.1 oz	90	16	15	3¾
Double Delights Low Fat Cheesecake Flavor w/ Chocolate Topping	8 oz	220	46	21	5¼
Double Delights Low Fat Cheesecake w/ Fruit, all fruit varieties	8 oz	160–180	33–37	30–33	7½–8¼
Fruit on the Bottom, low fat, all varieties	8 oz	210–250	43–46	40–45	10–11¼

FOOD	SERVING SIZE	CALORIES	CARBO-HYDRATES (GRAMS)	SUGAR (GRAMS)	SUGAR (TSPS)
Dannon (continued)					
Light Nonfat, all varieties, aspartame & fructose added	8 oz	120	21–23	15–20	4¼–5
Natural Flavors, low fat, all varieties	8 oz	220–230	37–36	35	8¾
Plain, full fat, whole milk (no sugar added)	8 oz	170	17	13	3¼
Plain, low fat (no added sugar)	8 oz	150	18	17	4¼
Plain, nonfat (no added sugar)	8 oz	130	19	17	4¼
Sprinkl'ins, all varieties	4.1 oz	110–130	21–24	19–20	4¾–5
Friendship					
Coffee	8 oz	210	30	29	7¼
Fruit Crunch, all varieties	6 oz	190	31–32	27–28	6¾–7
Plain, full fat	8 oz	150	13	12	3
Haagen Dazs					
all varieties, nonfat	½ cup	130–160	28–34	16–21	4–5¼
all varieties, low fat	½ cup	190	35	25	6¼
Hood					
Fat Free Plain	8 oz	130	18	18	4½
Fat Free, all varieties	8 oz	190	34–40	34–36	8½–9
Fat Free Swiss, all varieties	8 oz	210	45	40–41	10–10¼
Jell-O					
Low-fat, all varieties	4.4 oz	130	25	22	5½
La Yogurt					
French Style, Vanilla	6 oz	170	28	25	6¼
French Style, all other varieties	6 oz	180	32	29	7¼
French Style, nonfat, all varieties	6 oz	70–75	12–13	8	2
Latin Style, all varieties	6 oz	190	32–34	30–31	7½–7¾

FOOD	SERVING SIZE	CALORIES	CARBO-HYDRATES (GRAMS)	SUGAR (GRAMS)	SUGAR (TSPS)
Weight Watchers					
All varieties	8 oz	90	14	7–8	1¾–2
Yonique Drink					
Peach	6 oz	170	29	27	6¾
Pina Colada	6 oz	190	36	31	7¾
Strawberry	6 oz	190	36	31	7¾
Strawberry Banana	6 oz	140	28	27	6¾
Yoplait					
Custard Style, all varieties	6 oz	190	32	28	7
Light Yogurt, all varieties	6 oz	90	15–16	10	2½
Go-Gurt, all varieties	2½ oz	80	11	10	2½
Original, all varieties	6 oz	170–190	33–36	27–28	6¾–7
Trix Fruit Flavored	4 oz	120	23	18	4½
Frozen					
Ben & Jerry's					
Cherry Garcia	½ cup	170	31	30	7½
Chocolate Cherry Garcia	½ cup	170	32	27	6¾
Chocolate Chip Cookie Dough	½ cup	190	35	32	8
Chocolate Heath Bar Crunch	½ cup	210	35	30	7½
Chunky Monkey	½ cup	200	34	30	7½
Ooey Cookie Cake	½ cup	170	31	30	7½
Breyers					
Chocolate	½ cup	90–130	23	18	4½
Fat Free, all varieties	½ cup	90–110	20–25	15–18	3¾–4½
Colombo					
Cookies 'n Cream, nonfat	½ cup	120	25	22	5½
Low Fat, all varieties	½ cup	110–120	20–22	16–17	4–4¼

FOOD	SERVING SIZE	CALORIES	CARBO-HYDRATES (GRAMS)	SUGAR (GRAMS)	SUGAR (TSPS)
Colombo (continued)					
Nonfat, all other varieties	½ cup	100–110	20–23	16–17	4–4½
Slender Sensations, all varieties	½ cup	60–70	11	8	2
Dannon					
Light Cappuccino	½ cup	100	17	13	3¼
Light, all other varieties	½ cup	80–90	20–23	5–6	1¼–1½
Light 'N Crunchy	½ cup	90–110	23–25	11–13	2¾–3¼
Light Duets Strawberry Sundae	6 oz	90	18	12	3
Dreyer's					
all varieties	½ cup	100–140	17–23	13–18	3¼–4½
Fat Free, all varieties	½ cup	90–100	19–23	13–17	3¼–4¼
Friendly's					
Regular, all varieties	½ cup	130–160	21–25	15–21	3¾–4¼
Low Fat, all varieties	½ cup	110–120	19–21	15–17	3¾–4¼
Good Humor					
Creamsicle Raspberry	2.8 oz	100	23	22	5½
Frista Cup	6.2 oz	220	38	32	8
Haagen Dazs					
Chocolate Chocolate Chip	8 oz	230	32	26	6½
Coffee	8 oz	200	31	20	5
Strawberry	8 oz	140	31	20	5
Vanilla	8 oz	200	31	21	5¼

FOOD	SERVING SIZE	CALORIES	CARBO-HYDRATES (GRAMS)	SUGAR (GRAMS)	SUGAR (TSPS)

DESSERTS

See also Bakery and Dairy.

Pudding, Custard, and Pie Filling

The milk in pudding, custard, and pie filling contains the natural sugars galatose and lactose. You cannot tell from the label how much is added sugar and how much is natural.

Mix

FOOD	SERVING SIZE	CALORIES	CARBO-HYDRATES (GRAMS)	SUGAR (GRAMS)	SUGAR (TSPS)
Betty Crocker					
Flan	¼ cup	120	27	23	5¾
Rice Pudding	¼ cup	140	33	21	5¼
Cross & Blackwell					
Plum Pudding	⅓ of pkg	460	87	58	14½
Jell-O					
Cook & Serve					
Americana Custard Dessert, as prepared w/ milk	½ cup	140	25	23	5¾
Americana Rice, as prepared w/ milk	½ cup	140	29	19	4¾
Americana Tapioca, as prepared w/ milk	½ cup	130	28	21	5¼
Banana Cream, as prepared w/ milk	½ cup	140	26	21	5¼
Butterscotch, as prepared w/ milk	½ cup	160	30	25	6¼
Chocolate, as prepared w/ milk	½ cup	150	28	21	5¼

FOOD	SERVING SIZE	CALORIES	CARBO-HYDRATES (GRAMS)	SUGAR (GRAMS)	SUGAR (TSPS)
Cook & Serve (continued)					
Chocolate Fudge, as prepared w/ milk	½ cup	150	28	21	5¼
Coconut Cream, as prepared w/ milk	½ cup	150	24	19	4¾
Flan, as prepared w/ milk	½ cup	140	26	25	6¼
Lemon, as prepared w/ milk	½ cup	140	29	23	5¾
Milk Chocolate, as prepared w/ milk	½ cup	150	28	22	5½
Vanilla, as prepared w/ milk	½ cup	140	26	21	5¼
Gelatin Desserts					
all varieties, cook & serve	½ cup	80	19	19	4¾
Instant					
Banana Cream, as prepared w/ milk	½ cup	150	29	24	6
Butterscotch , as prepared w/ milk	½ cup	150	29	24	6
Chocolate, as prepared w/ milk	½ cup	160	31	25	6¼
Chocolate Fudge, as prepared w/ milk	½ cup	160	31	23	5¾
Coconut Cream, as prepared w/ milk	½ cup	160	27	22	5½
Fat-Free Devil's Food, as prepared w/ milk	½ cup	140	31	25	6¼
Fat-Free Vanilla, as prepared w/ milk	½ cup	140	29	25	6¼
Fat-Free White Chocolate, as prepared w/ milk	½ cup	140	29	25	6¼
French Vanilla, as prepared w/ milk	½ cup	150	29	24	6

FOOD	SERVING SIZE	CALORIES	CARBO-HYDRATES (GRAMS)	SUGAR (GRAMS)	SUGAR (TSPS)
Instant (continued)					
Lemon, as prepared w/ milk	½ cup	150	29	25	6¼
Milk Chocolate, as prepared w/ milk	½ cup	150	28	22	5½
Pistachio, as prepared w/ milk	½ cup	160	29	24	6
Vanilla, as prepared w/ milk	½ cup	150	29	25	6¼
Royal					
Chocolate Pie Filling	½ cup	90	23	18	4½
Flan	½ cup	70	18	17	4¼
Lemon Pie Filling	½ cup	80	21	17	4¼
Vanilla Cream Pie	½ cup	80	21	17	4¼

Ready to Eat

FOOD	SERVING SIZE	CALORIES	CARBO-HYDRATES (GRAMS)	SUGAR (GRAMS)	SUGAR (TSPS)
Comstock Pie Filling					
Apple Cranberry	½ cup	90	22	18	4½
More Fruit Apple	½ cup	90	23	18	4½
More Fruit Blueberry	½ cup	80	21	15	3¾
More Fruit Cherry	½ cup	90	23	18	4½
Red Ruby Filling	½ cup	90	23	19	4¾
Hunt's					
Pudding Pie					
Banana Cream	1 serving	140	22	17	4¼
Butterscotch	1 serving	130	21	15	3¾
Caramel Apple	1 serving	160	23	17	4¼
Chocolate	1 serving	140	22	17	4¼
Chocolate Mud Pie	1 serving	170	26	20	5
Chocolate Peanut Butter	1 serving	190	28	22	5½

FOOD	SERVING SIZE	CALORIES	CARBO-HYDRATES (GRAMS)	SUGAR (GRAMS)	SUGAR (TSPS)
Snack Pack					
Banana	3.5 oz cup	140	20	14	3½
Butterscotch	3.5 oz cup	130	21	14	3½
Chocolate	4.3 oz cup	140	22	17	4¼
Chocolate Fudge	3.5 oz cup	167	26	18	4½
Chocolate Vanilla fat free	3.5 oz cup	90	19	14	3½
Chocolate Marshmallow	3.5 oz cup	155	23	18	4½
Fat Free, all varieties	3.5 oz cup	90–96	19–21	14–17	3½–4¼
Lemon	3.5 oz cup	162	33	27	6¾
Swirl, all varieties	3.5 oz cup	154–160	25–26	19–21	4¾–5¼
Tapioca	3.5 oz cup	151	23	16	4
Vanilla	3.5 oz cup	130	21	17	4¼
Jell-O					
Pie Filling					
No Bake Chocolate Silk, as prepared	⅙ pie	320	27	20	5
No Bake Coconut Cream, as prepared	⅙ pie	330	27	26	6½
Pudding					
Chocolate	1 serving	160	28	23	5¾
Chocolate Marshmallow	1 serving	160	27	22	5½
Free Chocolate	1 serving	100	23	17	4¼
Free Chocolate Vanilla Swirl	1 serving	100	23	17	4¼
Free Devil's Food	1 serving	100	23	18	4½
Free Rocky Road	1 serving	100	23	17	4¼

*Jello-O instant sugar-free puddings do contain sugar in the form of sugar alcohol although the labels say that they are sugar free. A ½ cup serving has 6 grams or 1½ teaspoons of sugar.

FOOD	SERVING SIZE	CALORIES	CARBO-HYDRATES (GRAMS)	SUGAR (GRAMS)	SUGAR (TSPS)
Pudding (continued)					
Free Vanilla	1 serving	100	23	18	4½
Tapioca	1 serving	140	26	21	5¼
Vanilla	1 serving	160	25	21	5¼
Snacks					
Cheesecake Snacks Original	1 snack	160	23	19	4¾
Cheesecake Snacks Strawberry	1 snack	150	26	23	5¾
Fat-Free Pudding Snacks, all varieties	1 snack	100	23	17–18	4¼–4½
Gelatin Snacks, all varieties	1 snack	70	17	17	4¼
Pudding Snacks, all varieties	1 snack	140–160	25–28	21–23	5¼–5¾
Kozy Shack					
Chocolate	½ cup	150	26	20	5
Flan	½ cup	150	25	23	5¾
Rice cup	½ cup	140	24	18	4½
Tapioca	½ cup	150	27	22	5½
Vanilla	½ cup	140	24	19	4¾
Pudding Pack					
Banana	3.5 oz	119	18	14	3½
Butterscotch	3.5 oz	130	21	14	3½
Chocolate	3.5 oz	143	22	17	4¼
Chocolate Fudge	3.5 oz	147	23	17	4¼
Chocolate Marshmallow	3.5 oz	134	21	16	4
Chocolate Peanut Butter Swirl	3.5 oz	146	21	15	3¾
Lemon	3.5 oz	140	29	23	5¾

FOOD	SERVING SIZE	CALORIES	CARBO-HYDRATES (GRAMS)	SUGAR (GRAMS)	SUGAR (TSPS)
Pudding Pack (continued)					
Milk Chocolate	3.5 oz	143	22	18	4½
S'Mores	3.5 oz	136	21	18	4½
Vanilla	3.5 oz	135	21	17	4¼
Kraft					
Handi-snacks Gels, all varieties	1 snack	120–130	21–23	14–18	4½–5½
Handi-snacks Gels, all varieties, fat free	1 snack	90	21	17	4¼
Handi-Snacks Pudding, all varieties	1 snack	90–120	21–22	16	4
Libby					
Apple	1 cup	244	60	47	11¾
Pumpkin Pie Mix	1 cup	200	50	44	11
None Such					
Mincemeat Condensed	⅛ pkg	150	36	31	7¾
Mincemeat Ready-to-Use	⅓ cup	190	45	39	9¾
R & H Right Choice					
Peach	1 cup	294	74	53	11¾
S & W					
Snack Cups, all varieties	1 snack	140–160	25–27	19–20	4¾–5
Snack Cups, Lite, all varieties	1 snack	90–100	18–19	13–14	3¼–3½
Swiss Miss					
Butterscotch	4 oz	156	24	19	4¾
Chocolate Caramel Swirl	4 oz	169	26	20	5
Chocolate, fat free	4 oz	98	22	16	4
Chocolate Fudge	4 oz	175	28	22	5½
Chocolate Fudge, fat free	4 oz	101	23	17	4¼
Chocolate Sundae	3.5 oz	160	25	16	4

FOOD	SERVING SIZE	CALORIES	CARBO-HYDRATES (GRAMS)	SUGAR (GRAMS)	SUGAR (TSPS)
Swiss Miss (continued)					
Chocolate Vanilla Parfait, fat free	4 oz	160	24	22	5½
Tapioca	4 oz	120	21	15	3¾
Vanilla	4 oz	190	21	17	4¼
Vanilla Chocolate	4 oz	164	25	22	5½
Vanilla Sundae	4 oz	175	27	22	5½

Miscellaneous Desserts

FOOD	SERVING SIZE	CALORIES	CARBO-HYDRATES (GRAMS)	SUGAR (GRAMS)	SUGAR (TSPS)
Marie Callender's					
Apple Cobbler	4 oz	350	45	26	6½
Berry Cobbler	4 oz	390	41	29	7¼
Peach Cobbler	4 oz	370	47	24	6
Pepperidge Farms					
Apple Fruit Squares	2½ oz	210	27	20	5
Apple Puff Pastry	3 oz	290	44	32	8
Cherry Dumpling	3 oz	280	47	35	8¾
Peach Dumpling	3 oz	300	47	34	8½
Pet Ritz					
Apple Crumb Cobbler	4.4 oz	280	49	29	7¼
Blackberry Cobbler	4.4 oz	260	38	22	5½
Blackberry Crumb	4.4 oz	260	45	25	6¼
Blueberry Cobbler	4.4 oz	280	42	21	5¼
Cherry Crumb Cobbler	4.4 oz	280	54	30	7½
Peach Crumb Cobbler	4.4 oz	230	38	24	6
Strawberry Cobbler	4.4 oz	260	41	23	5¾
Weight Watchers					
Chocolate Eclair	1 eclair	150	25	14	3½
Chocolate Mousse	1 serving	190	31	6	1½

FOOD	SERVING SIZE	CALORIES	CARBO-HYDRATES (GRAMS)	SUGAR (GRAMS)	SUGAR (TSPS)
Weight Watchers (continued)					
Popcorn, Caramel and Butter Toffee	1 pkg	100	22	11	2¾

FRUIT

Whole fruit contains natural sugar. Some fruit is higher in sugar than others. Melons and berries contain the least, while dried fruit, because it is so concentrated, has the most sugar. Whole fruit also contains fiber, which slows the digestion process, making the nutrients easier to digest and metabolize. On the other hand, the sugar in fruit juice, because there is insufficient fiber to slow the process, enters the bloodstream much quicker, which can upset the body's chemistry. So, it's a good idea to eat your fruit whole.

As you will see under Canned Fruit, there is quite a difference between the sugar content of canned fruit with added sugar and the sugar content of canned fruit without added sugar. Interestingly, manufacturers are not required to state on the front label that sugar has been added to a product. It is only when sugar is *not* added that the manufacturer is required to state so on the front label. Of course this information is included in the ingredients on the nutrition label appearing on the back or side of the container.

You'll find that brand-name products are not listed in this section because the sugar content varies little from manufacturer to manufacturer. But always check the labels of the product you are buying.

See also Juice, Fruit, under Beverages and Jam, Jelly, Preserves, and Spreadable Fruit, under Sweeteners and Toppings.

FOOD	SERVING SIZE	CALORIES	CARBO-HYDRATES (GRAMS)	SUGAR (GRAMS)	SUGAR (TSPS)
Fresh					
Apple, unpeeled	1 med	81	21	18	4½
Apricots	3 med	51	11	10	2½
Banana	1 med	105	27	18	4½
Blackberries	1 cup	74	18	11	2¾
Blueberries	1 cup	81	21	11	2¾
Cantaloupe	¼ med	50	12	11	2¾
Casaba melon	1 cup cubes	44	11	9	2¼
Cherries	10 med	34	10	8	2
Elderberries	½ cup	53	13	8	2
Figs	1 med	74	19	14	3½
Grapefruit	½ med	40	10	7	1¾
Grapes, seedless	10 med	35	12	9	2¼
Honeydew melon	1/10 med	45	14	12	3
Jackfruit	3.5 oz	93	24	18	4½
Kiwifruit, without skin	2 med	92	22	8	2
Mango	1 med	135	35	31	7¾
Nectarine	1 med	67	16	12	3
Orange	1 med	60	18	16	4
Papaya	1 med	119	30	18	4½
Peach	1 med	37	10	8	2
Pear	1 med	98	25	17	4¼
Persimmon	1 sm	32	8	7	1¾
Pineapple	1 cup	76	19	18	4½
Plum	1 med	36	9	5	1¼
Pomegranate	1 med	105	27	21	5¼
Quince	1	52	14	12	3

FOOD	SERVING SIZE	CALORIES	CARBO-HYDRATES (GRAMS)	SUGAR (GRAMS)	SUGAR (TSPS)
Fresh (continued)					
Raspberries	1 cup	60	14	12	3
Strawberries	1 cup	45	11	9	2¼
Tangerine	1 med	37	9.	8	2
Watermelon	1 cup, diced	51	14	12	3
Canned or Jarred					
Applesauce, sweetened	1 cup	195	51	42	10½
Applesauce, unsweetened	1 cup	105	28	20	5
Apricots, fruit and liquid, heavy syrup	1 cup	215	55	52	13
Apricots, fruit and liquid, juice pack	1 cup	120	29	31	7¾
Blackberries, unsweetened	1 cup	120	26	6	1½
Cherries, dark, in heavy syrup	1 cup	200	48	48	12
Cherries	1 cup	90	25	24	6
Cranberry sauce, sweetened	¼ cup	110	28	27	6¾
Figs	3–4	110	26	20	5
Fruit cocktail, heavy syrup	½ cup	139	36	33	8¼
Fruit cocktail, juice pack	1 cup	120	29	29	7¼
Fruit cocktail, light syrup	1 cup	120	29	29	7¼
Grapefruit, unsweetened	1 cup	95	20	20	5
Mandarin oranges	1 cup	160	19	19	4¾
Papaya	¾ cup	120	29	29	7¼
Peaches, heavy syrup	1 cup	190	50	50	12½
Peaches, light syrup	1 cup	120	30	28	7
Peaches, juice pack	1 cup	124	30	28	7
Peaches, water pack	1 cup	60	15	12	3

FOOD	SERVING SIZE	CALORIES	CARBO-HYDRATES (GRAMS)	SUGAR (GRAMS)	SUGAR (TSPS)
Canned or Jarred (continued)					
Pears, heavy syrup	1 cup	200	48	46	11½
Pears, light syrup	1 cup	120	30	28	7
Pears, juice pack	1 cup	120	30	28	7
Pears, water pack	1 cup	71	19	15	3¾
Pineapple, heavy syrup	1 cup	180	48	44	11
Pineapple, juice pack	1 cup	140	34	30	7½
Pineapple, water pack	1 cup	78	20	19	4¾
Plums, heavy syrup	1 cup	250	60	53	13¼
Plums, juice pack	1 cup	145	38	32	8
Prunes, heavy syrup	½ cup	123	33	28	7
Raspberries, heavy syrup	½ cup	116	29	26	6½
Tangerines, light syrup	½ cup	155	20	19	4¾
Dried					
Apples, unsweetened	½ cup	73	20	16	4
Apples, sweetened	½ cup	116	20	25	6¼
Apricots	10 halves	83	21	13	3¼
Banana chips	½ cup	236	27	18	4½
Blueberries	¼ cup	140	33	17	4¼
Cherries	¼ cup	140	34	25	6¼
Currants	½ cup	202	53	49	12¼
Dates	10	228	61	53	13¼
Figs	10	477	140	124	31
Mango	6 slices (1.3 oz)	140	33	30	7½
Mixed Fruit	½ cup	165	44	38	9½
Papaya	2 pieces	200	41	35	8¾

FOOD	SERVING SIZE	CALORIES	CARBO-HYDRATES (GRAMS)	SUGAR (GRAMS)	SUGAR (TSPS)
Peaches	10 halves	311	80	58	14½
Pears	½ cup	236	63	47	11¾
Pineapple	2 slices	140	30	26	6½
Prunes	5 large	115	41	31	7¾
Prunes	½ cup	203	53	37	9¼
Raisins, seedless, not pressed down	½ cup	216	56	49	12¼
Raisins	½ oz	40	15	11	2¾

Frozen

FOOD	SERVING SIZE	CALORIES	CARBO-HYDRATES (GRAMS)	SUGAR (GRAMS)	SUGAR (TSPS)
Blackberries, unsweetened	⅔ cup	70	15	8	2
Blueberries, unsweetened	1 cup	80	20	16	4
Blueberries, sweetened	10 oz	230	62	62	15
Cantaloupe, unsweetened	¾ cup	40	10	7	1¾
Cherries, unsweetened	¾ cup	90	20	14	3½
Honeydew, unsweetened	¾ cup	45	11	7	1¾
Mixed Fruit	½ cup	122	32	28	7
Peaches, sliced	½ cup	118	30	28	7
Pineapple, chunks, sweetened	½ cup	104	27	25	6¼
Raspberries, unsweetened	⅔ cup	50	12	7	1¾
Raspberries, sweetened	½ cup	129	33	27	6¾
Strawberries, unsweetened	¾ cup	50	13	8	2
Strawberries, unsweetened, slices	½ cup	39	10	8	2
Strawberries, sweetened, sliced	½ cup	123	33	31	7¾

FOOD	SERVING SIZE	CALORIES	CARBO-HYDRATES (GRAMS)	SUGAR (GRAMS)	SUGAR (TSPS)

FRUIT SNACKS

Fruit snacks contain lots of sugar both in concentrated fruit form and added sugar form. There is a fine line between fruit snacks and candy. In fact, if you do not find a product you are looking for here, look under Candy. Remember, eat your fruit whole and fresh.

FOOD	SERVING SIZE	CALORIES	CARBO-HYDRATES (GRAMS)	SUGAR (GRAMS)	SUGAR (TSPS)
Betty Crocker					
Fruit by the Foot	1 roll	80	17	10	2½
Fruit Roll Ups	2 rolls	100	24	10	2½
Fruit Roll Ups XL Roll	2 rolls	130	28	12	3
Fruit Snacks	1 pouch	80	21	14	3½
Fruit Snacks XL Pouch	2 rolls	100	24	20	5
Fruit Snacks Mini Handouts	2 rolls	80	19	15	3¾
Fruit String Thing	1 pouch	80	17	9	2¼
Fruit Gushers	1 pouch	90	20	13	3¼
Fruitfield's Adult Fruit Shapes	10 pieces	100	23	15	3¾
Squeezit	1 bottle	110	24–29	23–26	5¾-6½
Squeezit 100	1 bottle	90	22	18	4½
Brock					
All varieties	1 pkg (0.9 oz)	90	21	14	3½
Favorite Brands					
Fruit Snacks, all varieties	1 pkg (0.9 oz)	80	19	14	3½
The Mega Roll Strawberry	1 pkg (1 oz)	110	22	14	3½
The Roll Cherry	1 pkg (0.75 oz)	80	16	10	2½
The Roll Strawberry	1 pkg (0.75 oz)	80	16	10	2½
Troll Fruit Snacks	1 pkg (0.9 oz)	80	19	14	3½
Zoo Animal Fruit Snacks	1 pkg (0.9 oz)	80	19	14	3½

FOOD	SERVING SIZE	CALORIES	CARBO-HYDRATES (GRAMS)	SUGAR (GRAMS)	SUGAR (TSPS)
Seneca					
Apple Chips	12 (1 oz)	140	20	11	2¾
Sensible Foods					
Crackin' Fruit Cherry Berry	1 pkg (0.6 oz)	51	14	13	3¼
Crackin' Fruit Tropical Fruit	1 pkg (0.6 oz)	65	16	14	3½
Stretch Island					
Fruit Leather, all varieties	2 pieces (1 oz)	90	24–25	21–26	5¼–6½
Sunbelt					
Fruit Boosters, all varieties	1 pkg (0.5 oz)	130	27	19–20	4¾–5
Fruit Jammers	1 (1 oz)	100	23	19	4¾
Weight Watchers					
Apple and Cinnamon	1 pkg (0.5 oz)	50	13	9	2¼
Apple Chips	1 pkg (0.75 oz)	70	18	13	3¼
Peach & Strawberry	1 pkg (0.5 oz)	50	13	11	2¾

MEALS, FROZEN AND REFRIGERATED

It's amazing how many frozen and refrigerated meals are available on today's market. It's impossible to include them all here. Also, many of them do not contain at least two teaspoons of sugar. On the other hand, many of them do. The most popular of these products are listed below. Note that children's frozen and packaged meals often have a high-sugar content. Once again, check your labels. (See "A Note about Frozen Meals" on page 143) Here are a few interesting facts to keep in mind: some meat packagers actually feed sugar to the animals to improve the flavor and color of cured meat; honey solutions are often injected into poultry before frying; and the breading on seafood often contains sugar.

FOOD	SERVING SIZE	CALORIES	CARBO-HYDRATES (GRAMS)	SUGAR (GRAMS)	SUGAR (TSPS)

(However, there are many manufacturers that produce fish, and seafood meals without additional sugar. Read labels before purchasing.)

Breakfast

FOOD	SERVING SIZE	CALORIES	CARBO-HYDRATES (GRAMS)	SUGAR (GRAMS)	SUGAR (TSPS)
Great Start					
French Toast w/ Sausage	5.6 oz	441	33	8	2
Pancakes w/ Bacon	4.5 oz	400	42	13	3¼
Pancakes w/ Sausage	6 oz	490	52	15	3¾
Swanson					
Great Starts Cinnamon Swirl	6 oz	440	34	11	2¾
Great Starts French Toast & Sausage	6 oz	410	33	8	2
Great Starts Pancakes & Bacon	5 oz	400	42	13	3¼
Great Starts Pancakes & Sausage	6 oz	490	52	15	3¾
Great Starts Silver Dollar Pancakes & Sausage	4 oz	340	36	11	2¾
Great Starts Sticks w/ syrup	4 oz	320	50	16	4

Children's Meals

FOOD	SERVING SIZE	CALORIES	CARBO-HYDRATES (GRAMS)	SUGAR (GRAMS)	SUGAR (TSPS)
Kids Cuisine					
Beef Pattie Sandwich	6.3 oz	270	40	22	5½
Cheese Pizza	7 oz	320	53	17	4¼
Chicken Sandwich	8.3 oz	440	63	25	6¼
Chicken Nuggets	8.6 oz	360	46	12	3
Fish Sticks	8.6 oz	340	54	26	6½
Fried Chicken	10.2 oz	440	48	11	2¾
Hamburger Pizza	7 oz	330	50	23	5¾

FOOD	SERVING SIZE	CALORIES	CARBO-HYDRATES (GRAMS)	SUGAR (GRAMS)	SUGAR (TSPS)
Swanson					
Blast Five Waffle Sticks	2.8 oz	330	39	32	8
Blast French Toast Sticks	3.8 oz	310	41	17	4¼
Blast Six Mini Pancakes	4.3 oz	320	54	24	6
Cheese Pizza	8 oz	350	57	27	6¾
Chomplin' Chic Drumlets	8 oz	490	51	19	4¾
Fish Sticks	7 oz	370	48	10	2½
Frazzlin' Fried Chicken	10 oz	580	53	17	4¼
Grilled Cheese Sandwich	6.6 oz	490	60	16	4
Meal Belly Bust, Beef Patties	8.1 oz	48	57	19	4¾
Spaghetti, Razzlin Rings	12 oz	390	60	33	8¼
Wobblin Wheels & Cheese	11.1 oz	370	59	28	7

Dinners

Beef

FOOD	SERVING SIZE	CALORIES	CARBO-HYDRATES (GRAMS)	SUGAR (GRAMS)	SUGAR (TSPS)
Banquet					
Beef Steak	10 oz	400	39	9	2¼
Chicken Fried	10 oz	800	73	14	3½
Meatloaf, Extra Helping	19 oz	650	49	13	3¼
Sliced Beef	9 oz	240	19	12	3
Healthy Choice					
Beef Macaroni	9 oz	210	34	9	2¼
Beef Meatloaf	11 oz	320	54	17	4¼
Beef Stroganoff	11 oz	310	44	21	5¼
Beef Tips	11 oz	260	32	18	4½
Charbroiled Beef Patty	11 oz	310	40	8	2

FOOD	SERVING SIZE	CALORIES	CARBO-HYDRATES (GRAMS)	SUGAR (GRAMS)	SUGAR (TSPS)
Healthy Choice (continued)					
Chili & Cornbread, Hearty Handful	1 bowl (10 oz)	340	49	13	3¼
Meatloaf	12 oz	330	52	17	4¼
Mesquite Beef w/ Barbecue Sauce	11 oz	320	38	16	4
Salisbury Steak	12 oz	330	48	24	6
Yankee Pot Pie	11 oz	290	38	25	6¼
Lean Cuisine					
Beef Macaroni	10 oz	280	40	9	2¼
Café Classics Country Vegetables & Beef	9 oz	200	31	9	2¼
Café Classics Southern Beef Tips	8.7 oz	270	37	10	2½
Hearty Portions Homestyle Beef Stroganoff	14 oz	350	44	12	3
Hearty Portions Salisbury Steak	15.5 oz	300	40	9	2¼
Skillet Sensations Savory Beef & Vegetables	24 oz	290	38	9	2¼
Marie Callender					
Beef Steak, fried w/ gravy	15 oz	650	69	9	2¼
Beef Pot Roast w/ noodles	13 oz	500	55	13	3¼
Meat Loaf	14 oz	540	42	30	7½
Salisbury Sirloin Steak & Gravy	14 oz	560	51	14	3½
Morton					
Meatloaf w/ tomato sauce	9 oz	250	24	17	4¼
Swanson					
Beef Meatloaf	11 oz	380	37	13	3¼
Beef Pot Roast	12 oz	250	39	15	3¾
Beef w/ Broccoli	10 oz	350	53	25	6¼

FOOD	SERVING SIZE	CALORIES	CARBO-HYDRATES (GRAMS)	SUGAR (GRAMS)	SUGAR (TSPS)
Swanson (continued)					
Beef w/ Gravy	11 oz	460	47	13	3¼
Beef w/ Noodles and Gravy	10 oz	290	34	15	3¾
Hungry Man Beef Pot Pie	14 oz	660	70	8	2
Hungry Man Chopped Beef	17 oz	620	44	32	8
Hungry Man Salisbury Steak	16.25 oz	690	41	12	3
Roast Beef Sandwich	10 oz	350	46	21	5¼
Weight Watchers					
Beef Macaroni	10 oz	220	32	15	3¾
Beef Meatballls	10 oz	280	35	8	2

A Note about Frozen Meals

When buying frozen meals, you may think that you're getting a nutritious dinner of meat, vegetables, pasta or potato, and fruit or dessert. What you may not realize is that there can be close to thirty ingredients or more contained in that seemingly simple meal, including preservatives, colorings, and hydrogenated oils and other difficult to digest substances. And what about the sugar content? In Hungry Man Salisbury Steak, for example, sugar appears on the ingredients list nine times in different forms! The long list of ingredients varies very little from package to package. So, next time you think about putting one of these frozen meals in your shopping cart, read the ingredients first.

Chicken

FOOD	SERVING SIZE	CALORIES	CARBO-HYDRATES (GRAMS)	SUGAR (GRAMS)	SUGAR (TSPS)
Banquet					
Chicken & Dumplings w/ gravy	10 oz	260	35	16	4
Chicken, BBQ style	9 oz	320	36	15	3¾
Chicken Nuggets	7 oz	410	38	11	2¾
Extra Helping Chicken Parmigiana	19 oz	650	64	9	2¼

FOOD	SERVING SIZE	CALORIES	CARBO-HYDRATES (GRAMS)	SUGAR (GRAMS)	SUGAR (TSPS)
Banquet (continued)					
Extra Helping Fried Chicken	18 oz	790	72	14	3½
Extra Helping Southern Fried	18 oz	60	67	14	3½
Extra Helping White Meat	18 oz	820	72	13	3¼
Green Giant					
Barbecue Chicken	½ cup	170	37	13	3¼
Garlic Herb Chicken	¾ cup	160	35	8	2
Healthy Choice					
Breaded Chicken Breast Strips	8 oz	270	34	9	2¼
Chicken, Country Breaded	10 oz	350	51	20	5
Chicken, Country Herb	12 oz	320	44	23	5¾
Chicken Cacciatore	12 oz	270	38	10	2½
Chicken Mesquite, BBQ	11 oz	310	48	13	3¼
Chicken Parmigiana	12 oz	330	46	23	5¾
Chicken Roasted	11 oz	230	25	9	2¼
Colonial Style Chicken Pie	10 oz	310	40	15	3¾
Country Glazed Chicken	9 oz	230	30	8	2
Grilled Chicken	9 oz	230	30	9	2¼
Sesame Chicken	10.8 oz	360	54	17	4¼
Lean Cuisine					
Café Classics Chicken a L'Orange	9 oz	230	33	9	2¼
Café Classics Chicken Parmesan	10.8 oz	300	41	8	2
Café Classics Chicken Piccata	9 oz	300	41	9	2¼
Café Classics Honey Mustard Chicken	8 oz	270	40	8	2

FOOD	SERVING SIZE	CALORIES	CARBO-HYDRATES (GRAMS)	SUGAR (GRAMS)	SUGAR (TSPS)
Lean Cuisine (continued)					
Café Classics Honey Roasted Chicken	8.5 oz	270	41	13	3¼
Chicken w/ Honey BBQ Sauce	9 oz	250	35	11	2¾
Chicken Honey Mustard	8 oz	250	32	12	3
Chicken Parmesan	10.5 oz	220	22	10	2½
Chicken Pot Pie	10 oz	320	39	13	3¼
Every Day Favorites Chicken Pie	9.5 oz	300	38	14	3½
Hearty Portions Chicken & BBQ Sauce	13.8 oz	370	60	31	7¾
Hearty Portions Glazed Chicken	13 oz	330	34	11	2¾
Skillet Sensations Herb Chicken & Roasted Potatoes	24 oz	270	39	10	2½
Skillet Sensations Three Cheese Chicken	24 oz	370	45	9	2¼
Marie Callender's					
Chicken & Dumplings	7 oz	260	22	8	2
Chicken & Gravy	1 cup	611	67	9	2¼
Chicken Parmigiana	16 oz	620	63	9	2¼
Chicken Pot Pie	10 oz	780	88	13	3¼
Fried Chicken & Gravy w/ Potatoes & Corn	16 oz	620	63	13	3¼
Grilled Chicken & Rice Pilaf	11.75 oz	360	38	14	3½
Morton					
Nuggets	7 oz	320	30	12	3
Patty, breaded	7 oz	280	24	12	3

FOOD	SERVING SIZE	CALORIES	CARBO-HYDRATES (GRAMS)	SUGAR (GRAMS)	SUGAR (TSPS)
Swanson					
Fried, Dark Meat	10 oz	580	54	17	4¼
Hungry Man Boneless White	15.5 oz	660	23	27	6¾
Hungry Man Fried	15.5 oz	790	75	19	4¾
Nuggets Platter	10 oz	590	71	32	8
White Fried Chicken Meat	11 oz	430	43	29	7¼
Tyson					
Chicken w/ BBQ & Tabasco	9 oz	320	36	15	3¾
Mesquite	9 oz	308	38	13	3¼
Mushroom Sauce	9 oz	218	28	8	2
Weight Watchers					
Chicken Lemon Herb Piccata	9 oz	190	32	8	2
Smart Ones Fiesta Chicken	8.5 oz	220	38	9	2¼
Smart Ones Honey Mustard Chicken	8.5 oz	200	37	10	2½
Smart Ones Lemon Herb Chicken Piccata	8.5 oz	200	34	8	2

Fish

FOOD	SERVING SIZE	CALORIES	CARBO-HYDRATES (GRAMS)	SUGAR (GRAMS)	SUGAR (TSPS)
Healthy Choice					
Herb Baked Fish	11 oz	340	54	11	2¾
Lemon Pepper Fish	11 oz	320	50	20	5
Shrimp Marinara	11 oz	250	44	27	6¾
Swanson					
Fish & Chips	10 oz	490	59	18	4½

Mexican Style

FOOD	SERVING SIZE	CALORIES	CARBO-HYDRATES (GRAMS)	SUGAR (GRAMS)	SUGAR (TSPS)
Banquet					
Chimichanga	10 oz	470	56	9	2¼

FOOD	SERVING SIZE	CALORIES	CARBO-HYDRATES (GRAMS)	SUGAR (GRAMS)	SUGAR (TSPS)
Healthy Choice					
Chicken Picante	11 oz	220	31	25	6¼
Enchilada Supreme	11 oz	300	46	8	2
Lean Cuisine					
Everyday Favorites Three Bean Chili w/ Rice	10 oz	250	39	8	2
Everyday Favorites Santa Fe-Style Rice & Beans	10 oz	300	54	10	2½
Swanson					
Beef Enchilada	14 oz	500	68	16	4
Hungry Man Mexican	20 oz	710	89	23	5¾
Mexican	14 oz	470	59	11	2¾

Oriental Style

FOOD	SERVING SIZE	CALORIES	CARBO-HYDRATES (GRAMS)	SUGAR (GRAMS)	SUGAR (TSPS)
Banquet					
Oriental w/ Egg Roll	9 oz	260	13	16	4
Green Giant					
Garlic & Ginger Stir Fry	¾ cup	130	25	14	3½
Sweet & Sour Stir Fry	½ cup	180	43	31	7¾
Szechuan Stir Fry	¾ cup	150	20	12	3
Teriyaki Stir Fry	¾ cup	100	18	10	2½
Healthy Choice					
Beef Broccoli Beijing	12 oz	300	45	11	2¾
Chicken Cantonese	11 oz	280	34	15	3¾
Chicken Ginger	12 oz	380	59	17	4¼
Chicken Teriyaki	11 oz	270	37	11	2¾
Mandarin Chicken	10 oz	280	44	9	2¼
Oriental-Style Chicken Stir Fry	11.9 oz	360	57	16	4
Sesame Chicken	10 oz	250	38	10	2½
Sweet & Sour Chicken	11 oz	360	53	25	6¼

FOOD	SERVING SIZE	CALORIES	CARBO-HYDRATES (GRAMS)	SUGAR (GRAMS)	SUGAR (TSPS)
LaChoy					
Chicken w/ Noodles	4 oz	196	19	15	3¾
Chicken Teriyaki	9 oz	110	15	9	2¼
Sweet & Sour Chicken	3 oz	180	29	10	2½
MuSho Pork	2 oz	191	25	8	2
Pork & Shrimp, mini	14 rolls	430	65	10	2½
Sweet & Sour Egg Rolls	2 oz	181	29	10	2½
Lean Cuisine					
Café Classics Oriental Beef	9 oz	210	30	8	2
Everyday Favorites Hunan Beef & Broccoli	8.5 oz	240	40	9	2¼
Everyday Favorites Mandarin Chicken	9 oz	240	36	8	2
Everyday Favorites Oriental Style Dumplings	9 oz	290	49	16	4
Everyday Favorites Teriyaki Stir-Fry	10 oz	290	45	9	2¼
Everyday Favorites Vegetable Egg Rolls	9 oz	300	57	16	4
Skillet Sensations Beef Teriyaki & Rice	24 oz	280	48	11	2¾
Skillet Sensations Chicken Oriental	24 oz	280	46	10	2½
Marie Callender's					
Chicken Sweet & Sour	14 oz	530	86	36	9
Swanson					
Sweet & Sour	12 oz	381	47	23	5¾
Weight Watchers					
Kung Pao Noodles & Vegetables	1 serving	250	37	12	3
Spicy Szechuan Style Vegetables & Chicken	1 serving	230	34	4	1

FOOD	SERVING SIZE	CALORIES	CARBO-HYDRATES (GRAMS)	SUGAR (GRAMS)	SUGAR (TSPS)
Pasta					
Banquet					
Chicken Pasta Primavera	10 oz	300	36	9	2¼
Lasagna w/ Meat Sauce	10 oz	260	35	10	2½
Green Giant					
Skillet Lasagna	¾ cup	150	31	10	2½
Healthy Choice					
Cheese Ravioli Parmigiana	9 oz	260	44	14	3½
Lasagna Primavera	7 oz	260	22	8	2
Macaroni & Cheese	9 oz	320	50	13	3¼
Macaroni w/ Three Cheeses	11 oz	300	40	14	3½
Pasta Italiano	10 oz	250	48	8	2
Potatoes Cheddar Broccoli	10 oz	330	53	8	2
Stuffed Pasta Shells	10 oz	370	60	12	3
Vegetable Pasta Italiano	10 oz	250	48	8	2
Zucchini Lasagna	14 oz	280	48	23	5¾
Lean Cuisine					
Everyday Favorites Angel Hair Pasta	10 oz	240	43	11	2¾
Everyday Favorites Cheese Cannelloni	9 oz	230	28	8	2
Everyday Favorites Cheese Ravioli	9 oz	260	38	8	2
Everyday Favorites Classic Cheese Lasagna	11.5 oz	290	88	9	2¼
Everyday Favorites Fettucini Primavera	10 oz	290	34	8	2
Everyday Favorites Penne Pasta w/ Tomato Basil Sauce	10 oz	260	47	13	3¼

FOOD	SERVING SIZE	CALORIES	CARBO-HYDRATES (GRAMS)	SUGAR (GRAMS)	SUGAR (TSPS)
Lean Cuisine (continued)					
Everyday Favorites Spaghetti w/ Meat Sauce	12 oz	290	50	10	2½
Everyday Favorites Vegetable Lasagna	11 oz	260	33	9	2¼
Hearty Portions Cheese & Spinach Manicotti	16 oz	370	50	14	3½
Hearty Portions Jumbo Rigatoni w/ Meatball	15 oz	440	65	12	3
Tuna Lasagna	10 oz	230	29	9	2¼
Marie Callender's					
Angel Hair Pasta w/ 2 oz breadstick	1 cup	460	60	9	2¼
Cheese Ravioli & Garlic Bread	16 oz	750	96	18	4½
Ham w/ macaroni & cheese	14 oz	450	63	32	8
Macaroni & Beef	14 oz	590	80	16	4
Weight Watchers					
Ravioli Florentine	9 oz	200	32	10	2½
Spaghetti w/ Meat Sauce	10 oz	250	24	10	2½
Tuna Noodle Casserole	9.5 oz	240	30	9	2¼

Pork

FOOD	SERVING SIZE	CALORIES	CARBO-HYDRATES (GRAMS)	SUGAR (GRAMS)	SUGAR (TSPS)
Healthy Choice					
Grilled Glazed Pork Patty	10 oz	300	44	28	7
Hearty Handful Ham & Cheese	6 oz	320	50	26	6½
Roasted Potatoes w/ Ham	9 oz	200	26	10	2½
Lean Cuisine					
Café Classics Honey Roasted Pork	10 oz	250	32	11	2¾

FOOD	SERVING SIZE	CALORIES	CARBO-HYDRATES (GRAMS)	SUGAR (GRAMS)	SUGAR (TSPS)
Swanson's					
Boneless Pork Rib	10.5 oz	470	58	28	7
Pork Patty	10 oz	470	58	28	7
Turkey					
Banquet					
Turkey Dinner, Extra Helping	19 oz	560	63	26	6½
Healthy Choice					
Country Inn Roast Turkey	10 oz	280	46	28	7
Hearty Handful Turkey & Vegetables	6 oz	320	51	10	2½
Traditional Breast of Turkey	11 oz	290	40	20	5
Turkey Roasted	10 oz	250	28	16	4
Lean Cuisine					
Café Classics Glazed Turkey Tenderloins	9 oz	240	37	19	4¾
Café Classics Roasted Turkey Breast	10 oz	270	49	27	6¾
Hearty Portions Roasted Turkey Breast	14 oz	320	43	11	2¾
Skillet Sensations Roasted Turkey	24 oz	220	37	10	2½
Turkey Pot Pie	9.5 oz	300	34	15	3¾
Swanson					
Turkey Breast w/ Pasta	11 oz	270	31	11	2¾
Turkey w/ mostly white meat	12 oz	330	42	15	3¾
Weight Watchers					
Smart Ones Stuffed Turkey Breast	10 oz	260	37	10	2½

FOOD	SERVING SIZE	CALORIES	CARBO-HYDRATES (GRAMS)	SUGAR (GRAMS)	SUGAR (TSPS)
Lunches					
Lunch Express					
Chicken Mandarin	10 oz	270	41	10	2½
Chicken Oriental	10 oz	320	45	12	3
Oriental Beef	10 oz	260	34	8	2
Rigatoni w/ Meat Sauce	10 oz	340	44	8	2
Teriyaki Stir Fry	10 oz	260	39	9	2¼
Turkey Dijon w/ Pasta	10 oz	270	37	8	2
Lunchables					
Bologna w/ Wild Cherry	11 oz	530	58	45	11¼
Chicken w/ Jack Cheese & Pudding	6 oz	370	33	16	4
Ham w/ American Cheese & Pudding	6 oz	390	34	17	4¼
Ham w/ Cheese & Vegetables	6 oz	380	36	13	3¼
Ham w/ Fruit Punch	11 oz	450	53	39	9¾
Ham w/ Herb Chive Cheese	6 Oz	390	37	14	3½
Turkey w/ Cheddar Cheese & Jello	6 oz	320	27	16	4
Turkey w/ Green Onion Cheese	4.5 oz	380	36	12	3
Turkey w/ Pacific Cooler	11 oz	460	53	38	9½
Turkey w/ Rice & Herb Cheese	4.5 oz	380	36	12	3
Miscellaneous					
Healthy Choice					
Pizza, all varieties	6 oz	280–340	44–51	7–9	1¾–2¼

FOOD	SERVING SIZE	CALORIES	CARBO-HYDRATES (GRAMS)	SUGAR (GRAMS)	SUGAR (TSPS)

MEALS, PACKAGED AND CANNED

FOOD	SERVING SIZE	CALORIES	CARBO-HYDRATES (GRAMS)	SUGAR (GRAMS)	SUGAR (TSPS)
Kraft					
Macaroni & Cheese Original, mix	1 cup	320	48	8	2
Macaroni & Cheese Thick & Creamy, mix	1 cup	320	50	9	2¼
Pasta Shapes & Cheese, mix	1 cup	390	48	8	2
Chef Boyardee					
ABC's & 123's	1 cup	200	43	12	3
Cheese Ravioli, 99% fat free	1 cup	240	45	9	2¼
Healthy Choice Overstuffed Beef Ravioli	1 cup	280	47	11	2¾
Homestyle Chicken Parmesan Style	1 cup	140	31	8	2
Homestyle Rigatoni	1 cup	250	31	8	2
Lasagna	1 cup	270	36	10	2½
Meat Tortellini	1 cup	270	45	12	3
Ravioli Primavera	1 cup	240	40	9	2¼

SALAD DRESSINGS

There are over 500 different types of salad dressing available. Many of them contain less than two teaspoons of sugar per serving. Watch out for the following salad dressings, which may contain two to three teaspoons of sugar per serving: Russian, French, honey mustard or any dressing with honey, fruit-flavored dressing, Oriental-style dressing, and coleslaw dressing.

FOOD	SERVING SIZE	CALORIES	CARBO-HYDRATES (GRAMS)	SUGAR (GRAMS)	SUGAR (TSPS)

SAUCES

Barbecue Sauce

There is a wide variety of barbecue sauces available from many different manufacturers. Popular BBQ sauce flavors include honey, honey mustard, honey smoked, hickory, mesquite, and spicy. They are all similar in sugar, carbohydrate, and calorie content, with approximately 45–70 calories, 10–13 grams carbohydrates, and 8–12 grams or 2–3 teaspoons of sugar per serving of two tablespoons. Hunts BBQ Honey Mustard and Hunts Hot and Spicy have the least amount of sugar with 6 grams or 1½ teaspoons, while Sweet Baby Reys has the most sugar with 16 grams or 4 teaspoons.

Cocktail Sauce

FOOD	SERVING SIZE	CALORIES	CARBO-HYDRATES (GRAMS)	SUGAR (GRAMS)	SUGAR (TSPS)
Heinz					
Cocktail Sauce for Seafood	3 tbsp	60	14	10	2½
Kraft					
Cocktail Sauce	¼ cup	60	13	9	2

Spaghetti and Pasta Sauce

Most spaghetti and pasta sauces have between 1½ and 2½ teaspoons of sugar per ½ cup serving. Read the labels.

SOUPS

There are very few soups that have more than two teaspoons of sugar per one cup, but there are a few exceptions. Soups prepared with milk have between 6 and 8 teaspoons of sugar due to the lactose in dairy, and soups containing tomatoes can have between 2 and 4 teaspoons of simple sugar from the tomatoes, and sometimes sugar may be added. Other exceptions are corn soup and bean soup, which can have between 4 and 6 teaspoons of sugar per serving. (When sugar comes from a product that contains fiber, such as corn and bean, the sugar is digested slowly and does not reach the bloodstream quick enough to upset the body's chemistry.) Also, some fat-free soups contain added sugar for flavor.

SWEETENERS AND TOPPINGS

As you've learned, there are four grams of sugar per teaspoon. However, some sweeteners are even more concentrated, and some are less concentrated, as you will discover below. For the majority of the products that you eat, four grams of sugar per teaspoon is the rule.

Baking Chips

Note that all semi-sweet and milk chocolate chips are between 3¾ and 4½ teaspoons sugar to two tablespoons of chips.

FOOD	SERVING SIZE	CALORIES	CARBO-HYDRATES (GRAMS)	SUGAR (GRAMS)	SUGAR (TSPS)
Hershey's					
Butterscotch	2 tbsp	164	20	18	4½
Mint Chocolate Chips	2 tbsp	156	20	18	4½
Raspberry	2 tbsp	160	20	18	4½
Skor English Toffee Bits	2 tbsp	134	15	14	3½
Vanilla Milk Chips	2 tbsp	160	19	19	4¾
Nestlé					
Peanut Butter Chocolate Chip	2 tbsp	170	19	12	3

FOOD	SERVING SIZE	CALORIES	CARBO-HYDRATES (GRAMS)	SUGAR (GRAMS)	SUGAR (TSPS)
Nestlé (continued)					
Rainbow Morsels	2 tbsp	130	21	16	4
White Morsels	2 tbsp	160	18	18	4½

Baking Chocolate

FOOD	SERVING SIZE	CALORIES	CARBO-HYDRATES (GRAMS)	SUGAR (GRAMS)	SUGAR (TSPS)
Chocolate, bittersweet	1 oz	140	14	10	2½
Chocolate, semi-sweet	1 oz	140	16	14	3½
Chocolate, sweet	1 oz	120	16	16	4
Chocolate, white	1 oz	160	17	17	4¼

Basic Sweeteners

FOOD	SERVING SIZE	CALORIES	CARBO-HYDRATES (GRAMS)	SUGAR (GRAMS)	SUGAR (TSPS)
Barley Malt	7 grams	20	5	3	1
Brown Sugar	4 grams	15	4	4	1
Confectioners Sugar	3 grams	10	3	3	1
Corn Syrup	6 grams	19	5	5	1
Fruit Juice Concentrate	7 grams	20	6	6	1
Granulated Cane Juice Sweetener	4 grams	15	4	4	1
High Fructose Corn Syrup	6 grams	20	5	5	1
Honey	7 grams	20	6	6	1
Maple Syrup	7 grams	15	4	4	1
Molasses	7 grams	20	5	5	1
Sucrose (table sugar)	4 grams	15	4	4	1
Rice syrup	7 grams	20	5	5	1
Sorghum Syrup	7 grams	20	5	5	1
Turbinado Sugar	4 grams	15	4	4	1

FOOD	SERVING SIZE	CALORIES	CARBO-HYDRATES (GRAMS)	SUGAR (GRAMS)	SUGAR (TSPS)

Dessert Frostings and Toppings

Ready to Spread

FOOD	SERVING SIZE	CALORIES	CARBO-HYDRATES (GRAMS)	SUGAR (GRAMS)	SUGAR (TSPS)
Betty Crocker					
Coconut Pecan	2 tbsp	160	21	18	4½
Creamy Deluxe Coconut Pecan	2 tbsp	140	17	16	4
Creamy Deluxe Party Frostings, all varieties	2 tbsp	140	22–24	20–23	5–5¾
Creamy Deluxe, all other varieties	2 tbsp	130–140	22–24	19–22	4¾–5½
Fluffy White	6 tbsp	100	24	23	5¾
Whipped Deluxe	2 tbsp	100	15	12–15	3–3¾
Betty Crocker Sweet Rewards					
All varieties	2 tbsp	120–130	24–27	22–25	5½–6¼
Kraft					
All varieties	2 tbsp	110–140	24–29	17–22	4¼–5½
Pillsbury					
Candy, Creamy	1.2 oz	150	22	20	5
Caramel Pecan	1.2 oz	149	19	16	4
Chocolate, Dark	1.2 oz	134	20	17	4¼
Chocolate Fudge	1.2 oz	135	21	18	4½
Chocolate Fudge, reduced fat	1.2 oz	135	27	23	5¾
Coconut Almond	1.2 oz	156	17	14	2½
Coconut Pecan	1.2 oz	160	17	14	2½
Cream Cheese	1.2 oz	147	24	22	5½
Funfetti	1.2 oz	128	20	18	4½
Lemon Creme	1.2 oz	146	23	21	5¼
Oreo	1.2 oz	144	23	21	5¼

FOOD	SERVING SIZE	CALORIES	CARBO-HYDRATES (GRAMS)	SUGAR (GRAMS)	SUGAR (TSPS)
Pillsbury (continued)					
Strawberry Creme	1.2 oz	146	24	21	5¼
Vanilla Funfetti	1.3 oz	155	25	23	5¾
Vanilla Pink Funfetti	1.2 oz	146	24	22	5½
Vanilla	1.3 oz	158	25	23	5¾
White	1.3 oz	127	21	18	4½
Glaze					
Marie's					
Banana	1.1 oz	40	9	9	2¼
Blueberry	1.1 oz	40	10	8	2
Peach	1.1 oz	40	10	8	2
Strawberry	1.1 oz	40	9	9	2¼
Pillsbury					
Chocolate Fudge	1.3 oz	140	22	18	4½
Vanilla w/ Fudge	1.3 oz	153	25	22	5½
Sprinkles					
Nestlé					
Buncha Crunch	0.7 oz	103	13	10	2½
Butterfinger	0.9 oz	120	16	12	3
Mini Morsels	0.7 oz	100	13	12	3
Rainbow Morsels	1 oz	136	21	17	4¼
Snow Caps Chocolate, Dark	1 oz	129	29	16	4

Flavoring and Sweetener for Milk

FOOD	SERVING SIZE	CALORIES	CARBO-HYDRATES (GRAMS)	SUGAR (GRAMS)	SUGAR (TSPS)
Powder					
Carnation					
Chocolate	4 tsp	110	24	20	5
Chocolate Malted	4 tsp	90	18	14	3½

FOOD	SERVING SIZE	CALORIES	CARBO-HYDRATES (GRAMS)	SUGAR (GRAMS)	SUGAR (TSPS)
Carnation (continued)					
Cocoa	1 pkt	70	15	15	3¾
Cocoa w/ marshmallows	4 tsp	110	24	21	5¼
Ghirardelli					
Double Chocolate Hot Chocolate	3 tbsp	80	19	17	4¼
Mocha Hot Chocolate	3 tbsp	80	18	16	4
Hershey					
Chocolate	3 tbsp	111	22	21	5¼
Ovaltine					
All flavors	4 tbsp	80	18	15	3¾
Swiss Miss					
Chocolate Flavor	5 tsp	145	28	24	6
Chocolate Flavor, lite	3 tsp	76	18	15	3¾
Milk Chocolate	4 tsp	118	22	16	4

Syrup

FOOD	SERVING SIZE	CALORIES	CARBO-HYDRATES (GRAMS)	SUGAR (GRAMS)	SUGAR (TSPS)
Estee					
Choco-Syp	2 tbsp	50	11	9	2¼
Hershey's					
Lite	2 tbsp	50	12	10	2½
Special Dark Chocolate	2 tbsp	110	27	22	5½
Strawberry	2 tbsp	100	25	25	6¼
Whoopers	2 tbsp	100	25	21	5¼
Marzetti					
Chocolate	2 tbsp	40	21	20	5
Quik					
Chocolate	2 tbsp	100	23	17	4¼
All other flavors	2 tbsp	130	24–25	22	5½

FOOD	SERVING SIZE	CALORIES	CARBO-HYDRATES (GRAMS)	SUGAR (GRAMS)	SUGAR (TSPS)

Ice Cream Toppings

FOOD	SERVING SIZE	CALORIES	CARBO-HYDRATES (GRAMS)	SUGAR (GRAMS)	SUGAR (TSPS)
Ben & Jerry's					
Chocolate Hazelnut Spread	1 tbsp	80	8	8	2
Hot Fudge	1.3 oz	140	19	8	2
Da Vinci					
Coconut	2 tbsp	170	39	20	5
Syrup, all varieties	2 tbsp	60	16	16	4
Hershey's					
Chocolate Syrup	2 tbsp	100	24	21	5¼
Chocolate Syrup, lite	2 tbsp	50	12	10	2½
Chocolate Malt Syrup	2 tbsp	100	25	21	5¼
Double Chocolate Fudge	2 tbsp	125	24	20	5
Double Chocolate Syrup, fat free	2 tbsp	113	25	16	4
Heath English Toffee Sundae Syrup	2 tbsp	100	24	19	4¾
Hot Fudge, fat free	2 tbsp	100	23	18	4½
Hot Fudge	2 tbsp	126	20	15	3¾
Strawberry Syrup	2 tbsp	100	26	26	6½
Kraft					
Butterscotch	2 tbsp	130	28	18	4½
Caramel	2 tbsp	120	28	19	4¾
Chocolate	2 tbsp	110	26	20	5
Hot Fudge	2 tbsp	140	24	17	4¼
Pineapple	2 tbsp	110	28	19	4¾
Strawberry	2 tbsp	110	29	22	5½
Marzetti					
Caramel Apple	2 tbsp	60	23	20	5

FOOD	SERVING SIZE	CALORIES	CARBO-HYDRATES (GRAMS)	SUGAR (GRAMS)	SUGAR (TSPS)
Marzetti (continued)					
Caramel Apple, reduced fat	2 tbsp	30	26	21	5¼
Peanut Butter Caramel	2 tbsp	60	21	14	3½
Nestlé					
Quik Chocolate Syrup	2 tbsp	100	23	17	4¼
Smucker's					
Ice Cream Topping Caramel	2 tbsp	130	31	21	5¼
Caramel Sundae Syrup	2 tbsp	110	25	19	4¾
Chocolate Magic Shell	2 tbsp	210	16	15	3¾
Hot Fudge	2 tbsp	140	24	16	4
Magic Shell	2 tbsp	200	19	11	2¾
Strawberry	2 tbsp	100	26	26	6½

Jam, Jelly, Preserves, and Spreadable Fruit

Jam, jelly, and preserves all contain added sugar, while spreadable fruit—which often contains concentrated fruit juice—does not. Smuckers offers six varieties of "fruit spreads." They are listed below for easy comparison with similar products. Your best choice here would be Smucker's Low Sugar even though it does contain added sugar. Although there is often more sugar than fruit in jams, jellies, and preserves, you won't find sugar listed as the first ingredient. This is because manufacturers divide the sugar content into two or more different ingredients and place them second, third, and so on on the label.

FOOD	SERVING SIZE	CALORIES	CARBO-HYDRATES (GRAMS)	SUGAR (GRAMS)	SUGAR (TSPS)
Generic					
Apple jelly	1 tbsp	52	14	12	3
Apple jelly	1 packet	38	10	9	2¼
Honey	1 tbsp	64	17	17	4¼
Jam, all varieties	1 tbsp	48	12–13	12–13	3–3¼

FOOD	SERVING SIZE	CALORIES	CARBO-HYDRATES (GRAMS)	SUGAR (GRAMS)	SUGAR (TSPS)
Generic (continued)					
Jam, all varieties	1 packet	34	9	7	1¾
Jelly, all varieties	1 tbsp	52	12–14	12–13	3–3¼
Jelly, all varieties	1 packet	38	10	9	2¼
Preserves, all varieties	1 tbsp	48	13	10	2½
Preserves, all varieties	1 packet	34	9	7	1¾
Spreadable Fruit, all varieties	1 tbsp	40	10	10	2
Smucker's					
Jelly	1 tbsp	50	13	12	3
Jam	1 tbsp	50	13	12	3
Light Sugar Free (Nutrisweet)	1 tbsp	10	5	0	0
Low Sugar	1 tbsp	25	6	5	1½
Preserves	1 tbsp	50	13	12	3
Simply Fruit, 100% Fruit	1 tbsp	40	10	8	2

Pancake and Waffle Syrup

FOOD	SERVING SIZE	CALORIES	CARBO-HYDRATES (GRAMS)	SUGAR (GRAMS)	SUGAR (TSPS)
Aunt Jemima					
Regular	¼ cup	212	53	38	9½
Butter Lite	¼ cup	209	52	29	7¼
Country Rich	¼ cup	212	53	30	7½
Country Rich, Lite	¼ cup	103	26	21	5½
Lite	1 packet	93	24	23	5¾
Country Kitchen					
Lite	¼ cup	100	26	25	6¼
All other varieties	¼ cup	200	53	40	10
Knotts Syrup					
All varieties	¼ cup	210	52	50	12½

FOOD	SERVING SIZE	CALORIES	CARBO-HYDRATES (GRAMS)	SUGAR (GRAMS)	SUGAR (TSPS)
Log Cabin					
Regular	¼ cup	200	53	40	10
Lite	¼ cup	100	26	25	6¼
Mrs Butterworth					
Original	¼ cup	230	56	35	8¾
Strawberry Flavored	¼ cup	220	55	39	9¾
Buttery Cinnamon	¼ cup	220	56	40	10
Mrs Richardson's					
Original Recipe	¼ cup	207	52	23	5¾
Hungry Jack Microwave Syrup					
Butter Maple	¼ cup	210	52	28	7
Butter Maple Lite	¼ cup	100	24	23	5¾
Regular	¼ cup	210	52	28	7
Regular Lite	¼ cup	100	24	23	5¾

VEGETABLES

All the vegetables in this section are high in starch, but surprisingly, not high in sugar and calories, as many people suspect. (They are included in this table to clear up this common misconception.) Sweet potatoes are the only vegetable that has more than two teaspoons of sugar per serving. But don't be fooled into thinking that vegetables with traditional toppings, such as glaze, sour cream, and butter, are healthy side dishes. Often the topping can have more calories and sugar than the vegetables themselves!

FOOD	SERVING SIZE	CALORIES	CARBO-HYDRATES (GRAMS)	SUGAR (GRAMS)	SUGAR (TSPS)
Fresh					
Beets, cooked	½ cup	37	9	6	1½
Carrot, uncooked	1 med	31	7	5	1¼

FOOD	SERVING SIZE	CALORIES	CARBO-HYDRATES (GRAMS)	SUGAR (GRAMS)	SUGAR (TSPS)
Fresh (continued)					
Corn, kernels	½ cup	89	21	2	½
Peas, uncooked	½ cup	58	10	4	1
Potato, baked w/ skin	7 oz	220	49	4	1
Sweet potato, baked w/ skin	½ cup	117	24	10	2½
Frozen					
Green Giant					
Corn on the Cob, Extra Sweet	1 med	120	22	13	3¼
Canned					
Green Giant					
Candied Sweet Potatoes	¾ cup	240	41	20	5
Harvard Beets	⅓ cup	60	15	10	2½
Honey Glazed Carrots	1 cup	90	13	10	2½
Three Bean Salad	½ cup	90	20	16	4
Mrs. Paul's					
Candied Sweet Potatoes	5 oz	300	73	47	11¾
Candied Sweet Potatoes w/ Applets	1¼ cup	270	66	47	11¾

Miscellaneous

FOOD	SERVING SIZE	CALORIES	CARBO-HYDRATES (GRAMS)	SUGAR (GRAMS)	SUGAR (TSPS)
Generic					
Beets, pickled w/ liquid, sliced	½ cup	79	19	16	4
Baked beans, canned	½ cup	170	30	10	2½
Cabbage, red, pickled	½ cup	110	29	28	7
Coconut, dried, sweetened, shredded	½ cup	233	22	16	4
Cranberry Sauce	½ cup	208	54	52	12
Ketchup	1 tbsp	16	4	4	1

FOOD	SERVING SIZE	CALORIES	CARBO-HYDRATES (GRAMS)	SUGAR (GRAMS)	SUGAR (TSPS)
Generic (continued)					
Peanuts and cashew mix, honey roasted	2 tbsp	300	20	10	2½
Pickle, sweet	1 med	41	11	10	2½
Tomato puree	½ cup	50	11	8	2

FAST FOODS

Many fast food companies were unable to provide all the nutritional information requested to provide you with a complete listing of all the fast foods available. However, the information below will give you a good idea of just how many calories and how much sugar you consume during a typical fast food meal. By the time you leave a restaurant, it's possible you've had more calories and sugar than you had imagined. For example, a typical meal from McDonalds may include a Big Mac (2¼ tsps of sugar), a salad with Red French Salad Dressing (3¾ tsps of sugar), and a medium Coke (14½ tsps of sugar). This meal delivers a whopping 20½ teaspoons of sugar—almost a half cup—and 930 calories! In all cases, beware of meal choices containing relatively small amounts of sugar in three or more different foods that collectively add up to a lot of sugar.

Many fast foods not mentioned, including bagels, soups, pizza, croissants, salad dressings, some chicken dishes, hamburgers, sandwiches, and casseroles, have one to two teaspoons of sugar. Interestingly, some restaurants add sugar, in the form of dehydrated molasses blended with corn syrup, to their hamburgers to reduce shrinkage.

Please note that the following fast food restaurants do not provide the nutritional information and/or sugar content of their products and are therefore not included in this section: Arby's, Bojangles, Captain D's,

FOOD	SERVING SIZE	CALORIES	CARBO-HYDRATES (GRAMS)	SUGAR (GRAMS)	SUGAR (TSPS)

Godfather's Pizza, Hardee's, Koo Koo Roo, Long John Silver, Papa John's, Red Lobster, Sizzler, Taco Time, and What a Burger.

Au Bon Pain

Bagel

FOOD	SERVING SIZE	CALORIES	CARBO-HYDRATES (GRAMS)	SUGAR (GRAMS)	SUGAR (TSPS)
Cinnamon Raisin	1	360	77	17	4¼
Chocolate Chip	1	380	69	14	3½
Dutch Apple w/Walnut Streussel	1	350	77	21	5¼
Onion	1	370	78	9	2¼
Sourdough					
Cranberry Walnut	1	460	93	19	4¾
Honey & Grain	1	360	72	9	2¼
Mocha Chip Swirl	1	370	72	13	3¼
Wild Blueberry	1	380	80	14	3½

Breakfast Sandwiches

FOOD	SERVING SIZE	CALORIES	CARBO-HYDRATES (GRAMS)	SUGAR (GRAMS)	SUGAR (TSPS)
All sandwiches	1	500–660	83	6–8	1½–2

Cookies

FOOD	SERVING SIZE	CALORIES	CARBO-HYDRATES (GRAMS)	SUGAR (GRAMS)	SUGAR (TSPS)
Almond	1	200	45	24	6
Chocolate Almond	1	240	28	13	3¼
Chocolate Chip	1	280	40	26	6½
Cranberry Almond Macaroon	1	160	22	19	4¾
English Toffee	1	220	28	16	4
Gingerbread Man Cookie	1	280	49	28	7
Ginger Pecan	1	260	30	15	3¾
Holiday Tree	1	200	36	23	5¾
Oatmeal Raisin	1	250	40	26	6½

FOOD	SERVING SIZE	CALORIES	CARBO-HYDRATES (GRAMS)	SUGAR (GRAMS)	SUGAR (TSPS)
Cookies (continued)					
Shortbread	1	390	39	13	3¼
Croissants					
Almond	1	560	50	19	4¾
Apple	1	280	46	19	4¾
Chocolate	1	440	53	25	6¼
Cinnamon Raisin	1	380	61	27	6¾
Raspberry Cheese	1	380	47	20	5
Danishes					
Cheese Swirl	1	450	46	18	4½
Lemon Swirl	1	450	53	21	5¼
Walnut Coffee Cake	1	480	50	22	5½
Desserts					
Apple Strudel	1	440	48	15	3¾
Cherry Strudel	1	450	45	17	4¼
Lemon Bar	1	440	54	31	7¾
Mochaccino Bar	1	380	56	34	8½
Oreo Cookie Bar	1	550	58	43	10¾
Southern Pecan Bar	1	560	60	43	10¾
Walnut Fudge Brownie	1	380	56	34	8½
Drinks					
Blasts, Hot, all flavors	16 oz	310–330	57	52	13
Frozen Mocha Blast	16 oz	320	64	58	14½
Iced Cappuccino, small	8 oz	110	10	10	2½
Iced Cappuccino, med	12 oz	150	15	15	3¾

FOOD	SERVING SIZE	CALORIES	CARBO-HYDRATES (GRAMS)	SUGAR (GRAMS)	SUGAR (TSPS)
Iced Cappuccino, large	16 oz	270	26	26	6½
Iced Tea, Peach, small	8 oz	90	22	22	5½
Iced Tea, Peach, med	12 oz	130	33	33	8¼
Iced Tea, Peach, large	16 oz	170	44	44	11
Malt Shoppe Blast	16 oz	370	71	60	15
Strawberry Banana Split Blast	16 oz	380	82	75	18¾
Muffins					
Blueberry	1	410	64	35	8¾
Carrot Pecan	1	480	61	34	8½
Chocolate Cake, low fat	1	290	68	43	10¾
Chocolate Chip	1	490	70	34	8½
Corn	1	470	70	30	7½
Pumpkin w/ streusel topping	1	470	74	37	9¼
Raisin Bran	1	390	66	43	10¾
Triple Berry, low fat	1	270	60	28	7
Rolls					
Cinnamon	1	340	48	13	3¼
Pecan	1	900	111	61	15¼
Salad					
Chicken Tarragon w/ Almonds	1	470	38	8	2
Garden, Large	1	160	34	8	2
Oriental Chicken	1	270	17	8	2
Thai Chicken (dressing below)	1	330	23	8	2
Tuna	1	490	40	9	2¼

FOOD	SERVING SIZE	CALORIES	CARBO-HYDRATES (GRAMS)	SUGAR (GRAMS)	SUGAR (TSPS)
Salad Dressing					
Fat-Free Tomato Basil	3 oz	70	17	13	3¼
Lite Italian	3 oz	230	15	14	3½
Thai Peanut Dressing	2 oz	130	16	12	3

Sandwiches

All other sandwiches have between 1¼ and 3 teaspoons of sugar.

FOOD	SERVING SIZE	CALORIES	CARBO-HYDRATES (GRAMS)	SUGAR (GRAMS)	SUGAR (TSPS)
Honey Smoked Turkey	1	540	89	15	3¾

Soup

Most Au Bon Pain soups come in three sizes. The 8 oz size soup has about 1 teaspoon of sugar. The 12 oz size has between 1½ to 2½ teaspoons of sugar. The 16 oz size has between 2½ to 3½ teaspoons of sugar.

FOOD	SERVING SIZE	CALORIES	CARBO-HYDRATES (GRAMS)	SUGAR (GRAMS)	SUGAR (TSPS)
Yogurt					
Blueberry w/ Fresh Berries	8.5 oz	210	42	37	9¼
Blueberry w/ Granola	8 oz	230	45	37	9¼
Plain w/ Fresh Berries	8.5 oz	210	38	33	8¼
Plain w/ Granola	8 oz	230	41	33	8¼
Strawberry w/ Fresh Berries	8.5 oz	210	42	37	9¼
Strawberry w/ Granola	8 oz	230	45	37	9¼

Baskin Robbins

FOOD	SERVING SIZE	CALORIES	CARBO-HYDRATES (GRAMS)	SUGAR (GRAMS)	SUGAR (TSPS)
Blasts					
Cappuccino w/ whipped cream	1 cup	160	22	22	5½
Cappuccino, nonfat	1 cup	90	20	16	4
Chocolate w/ whipped cream	1 cup	250	46	20	5
Chocolate, nonfat	1 cup	170	40	12	3
Mocca Cappy w/ whipped cream	1 cup	180	28	19	4¾

FOOD	SERVING SIZE	CALORIES	CARBO-HYDRATES (GRAMS)	SUGAR (GRAMS)	SUGAR (TSPS)
Blasts (continued)					
Mocha Cappuccino, nonfat	1 cup	120	26	13	4¼
Pina Colada	1 cup	190	33	30	7½
Pina Colada w/ whipped cream	1 cup	200	33	30	7½
Pina Colada, nonfat	1 cup	140	31	25	6¼
FroZone Kids Flavors					
Dirt 'N Worms	½ cup	160	22	19	4¾
Eerie I Scream	½ cup	150	18	17	4¼
Neon Sour Apple Ice	½ cup	110	27	27	6¾
Polar Paws	½ cup	160	17	16	4
Pink Bubblegum	½ cup	150	19	15	3¾
Skullicious	½ cup	170	18	17	4¼
Watermelon Ice	½ cup	110	28	28	7
Ice Cream, nonfat and low fat					
Espresso 'N Cream, low fat	½ cup	100	18	16	4
Nonfat, all flavors	½ cup	100–110	21–24	19–22	4¾–5½
Ice Cream (permanent flavors)					
Chocolate	½ cup	150	18	16	4
Chocolate Chip	½ cup	150	15	14	3½
Chocolate Chip Cookie Dough	½ cup	170	20	16	4
Chocolate Fudge	½ cup	160	21	19	4¾
Cookies & Cream	½ cup	170	16	14	3½
French Vanilla	½ cup	160	14	14	3½
Gold Medal Ribbon	½ cup	150	20	19	4¾
Jamoca	½ cup	140	14	14	3½
Jamoca Almond Fudge	½ cup	160	17	16	4

FOOD	SERVING SIZE	CALORIES	CARBO-HYDRATES (GRAMS)	SUGAR (GRAMS)	SUGAR (TSPS)
Ice Cream (permanent flavors) (continued)					
Mint Chocolate Chip	½ cup	150	15	14	3½
Old Fashion Butter Pecan	½ cup	160	13	12	3
Peanut Butter 'N Chocolate	½ cup	180	16	15	3¾
Pistachio Almond	½ cup	170	13	12	4
Pralines 'N Cream	½ cup	160	19	18	4½
Rocky Road	½ cup	170	19	17	4¼
Vanilla	½ cup	140	14	14	3½
Very Berry Strawberry	½ cup	130	16	15	3¾
World Class Chocolate	½ cup	160	18	17	4¼
Ice Cream (Rotating Flavors)					
Banana Strawberry	½ cup	130	17	16	4
Baseball Nut	½ cup	160	18	17	4¼
Black Walnut	½ cup	160	13	12	3
Blueberry Cheesecake	½ cup	150	18	17	4¼
Cherries Jubilee	½ cup	140	16	14	3½
Chocolate Almond	½ cup	180	17	15	3¾
Chocolate Mousse Royale	½ cup	170	20	18	4½
Chocolate Raspberry Truffle	½ cup	180	23	21	5¼
Chunky Heath Bar	½ cup	170	19	18	4½
Egg Nog	½ cup	150	16	16	4
English Toffee	½ cup	160	19	18	4½
Everybody's Favorite Candy Bar	½ cup	170	20	19	4¾
Fudge Brownie	½ cup	170	19	19	4¾
German Chocolate Cake	½ cup	180	20	19	4¾

FOOD	SERVING SIZE	CALORIES	CARBO-HYDRATES (GRAMS)	SUGAR (GRAMS)	SUGAR (TSPS)
Ice Cream (Rotating Flavors) (continued)					
Lemon Custard	½ cup	150	16	16	4
Mississippi Mud	½ cup	160	22	20	5
Oregon Blackberry	½ cup	140	16	14	3½
Pumpkin Pie	½ cup	130	16	15	3¾
Quarterback Crunch	½ cup	160	18	17	4¼
Reese's Peanut Butter	½ cup	180	17	16	4
Rum Raisin	½ cup	140	18	18	4½
Strawberry Shortcake	½ cup	160	18	16	4
Tripple Chocolate Passion	½ cup	180	21	18	4½
Winter White Chocolate	½ cup	150	18	16	4
Sherbert, Sorbet, and Ices					
Ices, all flavors	½ cup	110	27–29	27–28	6¾–7
Sherbert, all flavors	½ cup	120	22–26	21–25	5¼–6¼
Sorbet, all flavors	½ cup	120	29–31	27–29	6¾–7¼
Smoothies					
Aloha Berry Banana	16 fl oz	320	71	61	15¼
Berries Gone Bananas	16 fl oz	400	89	79	19¾
Just Peachy	16 fl oz	280	60	55	14¾
Orange Banana	16 fl oz	140	30	19	4¾
Orange Raspberry Banana	16 fl oz	170	38	33	8¼
Strawberry Banana	16 fl oz	180	40	28	7
Tropical Blueberry	16 fl oz	160	36	25	6¼
Tropical Raspberry Blueberry	16 fl oz	190	44	40	10
Very Strawberry	16 fl oz	370	81	74	18½

FOOD	SERVING SIZE	CALORIES	CARBO-HYDRATES (GRAMS)	SUGAR (GRAMS)	SUGAR (TSPS)

Blimpies

Blimpies sandwiches have between one and two teaspoons of sugar.

Boston Market

Baked Goods

FOOD	SERVING SIZE	CALORIES	CARBO-HYDRATES (GRAMS)	SUGAR (GRAMS)	SUGAR (TSPS)
Corn Bread	1 loaf	200	33	13	3¼
Cinnamon Apple Pie	⅙ pie	390	46	22	5½
Chocolate Chip Cookie	1 cookie	340	48	29	7¼
Brownie	1 piece	450	47	32	8

Entrees

FOOD	SERVING SIZE	CALORIES	CARBO-HYDRATES (GRAMS)	SUGAR (GRAMS)	SUGAR (TSPS)
Tabasco BBQ Drumstick	2 pieces	260	8	8	2
Tabasco BBQ Wings	2 pieces	220	8	8	2
Teriyaki Chicken, dark & white	¼ whole	340–380	17	14–15	3½–3¾

Sandwiches

FOOD	SERVING SIZE	CALORIES	CARBO-HYDRATES (GRAMS)	SUGAR (GRAMS)	SUGAR (TSPS)
BBQ Chicken Sandwich	1	540	84	33	8¼
Chicken Sandwich w/ cheese & sauce	1	750	72	13	3¼
Chicken Sandwich w/o cheese or sauce	1	430	62	12	3
Ham Sandwich w/ cheese & sauce	1	750	72	20	5
Ham Sandwich w/o cheese or sauce	1	440	66	16	4
Meat Loaf Sandwich w/ cheese	1	860	95	21	5¼
Meat Loaf Sandwich w/o cheese	1	690	86	21	5¼

FOOD	SERVING SIZE	CALORIES	CARBO-HYDRATES (GRAMS)	SUGAR (GRAMS)	SUGAR (TSPS)
Sandwiches (continued)					
Open Faced Meat Loaf Sandwich	1	760	71	10	2½
Open Faced Turkey Sandwich	1	500	61	13	3¼
Pastry Sandwich, BBQ Chicken	1	640	56	13	3¼
Turkey Sandwich w/ cheese and sauce	1	710	68	17	4¼
Turkey Sandwich, w/o cheese or sauce	1	400	61	12	3
Side Dishes, cold					
Cranberry Relish	¾ cup	370	84	72	18
Chunky Cinnamon Apple Sauce	¾ cup	250	62	58	14½
Cole Slaw	¾ cup	300	30	26	6½
Fruit Salad	¾ cup	70	15	14	4½
Old-Fashioned Potato Salad	¾ cup	340	30	8	2
Side Dishes, hot					
Baked Sweet Potato	1 med	460	94	49	12¼
BBQ Baked Beans	¾ cup	270	48	20	5
Butternut Squash	¾ cup	160	25	13	3¼
Cinnamon Apples	¾ cup	250	56	48	12
Honey Glazed Carrots	¾ cup	280	35	9	2¼
Macaroni & Cheese	¾ cup	280	32	8	2
Squash Casserole	¾ cup	330	20	8	2
Sweet Potato Casserole	¾ cup	280	39	23	5¾
Whole Kernel Corn	¾ cup	180	30	13	3¼

FOOD	SERVING SIZE	CALORIES	CARBO-HYDRATES (GRAMS)	SUGAR (GRAMS)	SUGAR (TSPS)
Soups and Salads					
Tomato Bisque	1 cup	280	16	12	3
Tossed Salad, individual w/ fat-free dressing	1 serving	160	29	9	2¼

Burger King

FOOD	SERVING SIZE	CALORIES	CARBO-HYDRATES (GRAMS)	SUGAR (GRAMS)	SUGAR (TSPS)
Burgers and Sandwiches					
Chicken Sandwich Broiler	1	530	45	29	7¼
French Toast Sticks	5	440	51	12	3
Whopper	1	680	47	8	2
Whopper, Double	1	920	47	8	2
Whopper, Double w/ Cheese	1	1010	47	8	2
Whopper w/ cheese	1	760	47	8	2
Desserts					
Cini-minis (4 rolls) w/o icing	1	440	51	20	5
Dutch Apple Pie	1	300	38	22	5½
Shakes					
Chocolate, small	10.8 fl oz	330	58	51	12¾
Chocolate w/ added syrup, small	11.8 fl oz	390	72	66	14
Chocolate, med	14.1 fl oz	440	75	76	19
Chocolate w/ added syrup, med	16.2 fl oz	570	105	96	24
Strawberry w/ added syrup, small	11.8 fl oz	390	72	66	14
Strawberry w/ added syrup, med	16.2 fl oz	540	105	96	24
Vanilla, small	10.8 fl oz	330	56	51	12¾
Vanilla, med	14 fl oz	430	73	66	16½

FOOD	SERVING SIZE	CALORIES	CARBO-HYDRATES (GRAMS)	SUGAR (GRAMS)	SUGAR (TSPS)

Carl's Jr.

Burgers and Sandwiches

FOOD	SERVING SIZE	CALORIES	CARBO-HYDRATES (GRAMS)	SUGAR (GRAMS)	SUGAR (TSPS)
BBQ Chicken	1	280	37	9	2¼
Famous Star Hamburger	9 oz	580	49	10	2½
Jacks Spicy Chicken	1	570	52	9	2¼
Super Star Hamburger	12.3 oz	790	50	10	2½
Western Double Bacon Cheeseburger	8 oz	650	63	16	4
Double Western Bacon Cheeseburger	11 oz	900	64	16	4

Breakfast

FOOD	SERVING SIZE	CALORIES	CARBO-HYDRATES (GRAMS)	SUGAR (GRAMS)	SUGAR (TSPS)
Cheese Danish	1 danish	400	49	21	5¼
French Toast Dips	3.5 oz	370	42	11	2¾
Table Syrup	1 packet	300	49	27	6¾

Desserts

FOOD	SERVING SIZE	CALORIES	CARBO-HYDRATES (GRAMS)	SUGAR (GRAMS)	SUGAR (TSPS)
Chocolate Cake	1 piece	300	49	27	6¾
Chocolate Chip Cookie	1 piece	370	49	29	7¼
Strawberry Swirl Cheesecake	1 piece	290	30	20	5

Salad Dressing

FOOD	SERVING SIZE	CALORIES	CARBO-HYDRATES (GRAMS)	SUGAR (GRAMS)	SUGAR (TSPS)
Fat-Free French Dressing	1 pkg	60	16	12	3
Thousand Island Dressing	1 pkg	230	16	12	3

Chick-fil-A

Beverages

FOOD	SERVING SIZE	CALORIES	CARBO-HYDRATES (GRAMS)	SUGAR (GRAMS)	SUGAR (TSPS)
Coca-Cola Classic	9 fl oz	255	28	28	7
Iced Tea, sweetened	9 fl oz	255	38	38	9½

FOOD	SERVING SIZE	CALORIES	CARBO-HYDRATES (GRAMS)	SUGAR (GRAMS)	SUGAR (TSPS)
Beverages (continued)					
Lemonade	9 fl oz	255	23	22	5½
Desserts					
Cheesecake, slice	3.1 oz	270	7	5	1¼
Cheesecake, slice, strawberry & blueberry topping	4.1 oz	290	8–9	6	1½
Fudge Nut Brownie	2.6 oz	350	41	37	9¼
Icedream, small cone	4.5 oz	140	16	16	4
Icedream, small cup	7.5 oz	350	50	38	9½
Lemon Pie, slice	4.0 oz	320	40	25	6¼
Salads					
Chicken-n-Strips Salad	1	370	21	7	1¾
Sauces					
Barbeque Sauce	1	45	11	9	2¼
Honey Mustard Sauce	1	45	11	10	2½
Polynesian Sauce	1	110	13	12	3

Church's Fried Chicken

FOOD	SERVING SIZE	CALORIES	CARBO-HYDRATES (GRAMS)	SUGAR (GRAMS)	SUGAR (TSPS)
Apple Pie	1	280	41	13	3¼

Dairy Queen

FOOD	SERVING SIZE	CALORIES	CARBO-HYDRATES (GRAMS)	SUGAR (GRAMS)	SUGAR (TSPS)
Blizzard Flavor Treats					
Choc. Chip Cookie Dough, small	11.1 oz	660	99	74	18½
Choc. Chip Cookie Dough, med	15.6 oz	950	143	106	26½
Choc. Sandwich Cookie, small	9.8 oz	520	79	61	15¼

FOOD	SERVING SIZE	CALORIES	CARBO-HYDRATES (GRAMS)	SUGAR (GRAMS)	SUGAR (TSPS)
Blizzard Flavor Treats (continued)					
Choc. Sandwich Cookie, med	11.6 oz	640	97	74	18½
Cones					
Chocolate, small	5 oz	240	37	25	6¼
Chocolate, med	7 oz	340	53	34	8½
Chocolate Soft Serve	½ cup	150	22	17	4¼
Dipped, small	5.5 oz	340	42	31	7¾
Dipped, med	7.8 oz	490	59	43	10¾
Vanilla, small	5 oz	230	38	27	6¾
Vanilla, med	7 oz	330	53	38	9½
Vanilla, large	9 oz	410	65	49	12½
Vanilla Soft Serve	½ cup	140	22	19	4¾
Frozen Yogurt					
Frozen, nonfat	3 oz	100	21	16	4
Heath Breeze, small	10 oz	470	85	70	17½
Heath Breeze, med	14.5 oz	710	123	103	25¾
Strawberry Breeze, small	9.5 oz	320	68	54	13½
Strawberry Breeze, med	13.6 oz	460	99	79	19¾
Strawberry Sundae, med	8.3 oz	280	61	49	12¼
Whole Fat, med	7 oz	260	56	36	9
Malts, Shakes, Smoothys, and Misty Slushes					
Chocolate Malt, small	15 oz	650	111	95	23¾
Chocolate Malt, med	20 oz	888	153	131	32¾
Chocolate Shake, small	14 oz	560	94	81	20¼
Chocolate Shake, med	19 oz	770	130	113	28¼

FOOD	SERVING SIZE	CALORIES	CARBO-HYDRATES (GRAMS)	SUGAR (GRAMS)	SUGAR (TSPS)
Malts, Shakes, Smoothys, and Misty Slushes (continued)					
Frozen Hot Chocolate	21 oz	860	127	109	27¼
Misty Slush, small	16 oz	220	56	56	14
Misty Slush, med	21 oz	290	74	74	18½
Strawberry Banana Glacier Smoothy	22 oz	670	128	114	28½
Novelties					
Bustar Bar	5.3 oz	450	41	33	8¼
Chocolate Dilly Bar	3.0 oz	210	21	17	4¼
Ice Cream Sandwich	2.1 oz	150	24	13	3¼
Lemon Freeze	3.2 oz	80	20	20	5
Starkiss	3.0 oz	80	21	21	5¼
Royal Treats					
Banana Split	13 oz	510	96	82	20½
Chocolate Rock Treat	10 oz	730	87	74	18½
Peanut Buster Parfait	11 oz	730	99	85	21¼
Pecan Mudslide Treat	5 oz	650	85	70	17½
Strawberry Shortcake	7 oz	430	70	57	14¼
Sundaes					
Chocolate Sundae, small	6 oz	280	49	42	10½
Chocolate Sundae, med	8 oz	400	71	61	15¼

Del Taco

FOOD	SERVING SIZE	CALORIES	CARBO-HYDRATES (GRAMS)	SUGAR (GRAMS)	SUGAR (TSPS)
Burritos, Salads, and Sides					
Beans & Cheese Cup	7.8 oz	260	44	16	4
Burrito, all types	19.2 oz	1,170	89	8	2

FOOD	SERVING SIZE	CALORIES	CARBO-HYDRATES (GRAMS)	SUGAR (GRAMS)	SUGAR (TSPS)
Burritos, Salads, and Sides (continued)					
Deluxe Taco Salad	19.3 oz	780	76	9	2¼
Deluxe Chicken Salad	18.7 oz	730	75	8	2
Macho Burrito, all types	19.7 oz	1,050	113	9	4¼
Get A Lot Meal					
#1 Combo Burrito, Fries, Drink	27.3 oz	1,020	132	41	10¼
#2 Del Classic Chicken Burrito, Fries, Drink	25.8 oz	1,050	112	41	10¼
#3 Chicken Quesadilla, Fries, Drink	24.6 oz	1,070	111	40	10
#4 Two Chicken Soft Tacos, Fries, Drink	85.5 oz	910	101	39	9¾
#5 Deluxe Del Beef Burrito, Fries, Drink	99.7 oz	1,080	115	42	10½
#6 Two Tacos, Quesadilla, Drink	22.5 oz	960	98	40	10
#7 Macho Combo Burrito, Fries, Drink	37.4 oz	1,540	183	47	11¾
#8 Two Big Fat Tacos, Fries, Drink	28.6 oz	1,130	148	44	11
#9 Double Del Deluxe Cheeseburger, Fries, Drink	24.9 oz	1,050	106	41	10¼
Shakes					
Chocolate Shake, small	1 serving	520	89	77	19¼
Chocolate Shake, large	1 serving	680	111	101	25¼
Strawberry Shake, small	1 serving	410	76	65	16¼
Strawberry Shake, large	1 serving	540	100	85	21¼
Vanilla Shake, small	1 serving	420	75	62	15½

FOOD	SERVING SIZE	CALORIES	CARBO-HYDRATES (GRAMS)	SUGAR (GRAMS)	SUGAR (TSPS)
Shakes (continued)					
Vanilla Shake, large	1 serving	505	97	81	20¼

Domino's Pizza

There are about 1½ to 2 teaspoons of sugar in each serving of Domino pizza.

Dunkin' Donuts

FOOD	SERVING SIZE	CALORIES	CARBO-HYDRATES (GRAMS)	SUGAR (GRAMS)	SUGAR (TSPS)
Bagels and Croissants					
Almond Croissant, USA	1 croissant	350	34	13	3¼
Chocolate Croissant, USA	1 croissant	400	37	15	3¾
Cinnamon Raisin Bagel	1 bagel	340	74	11	2¾
Cookies					
Chocolate Chocolate Chunk	1 cookie	210	26	16	4
Chocolate Chunk	1 cookie	220	28	17	4½
Chocolate Chunk w/ Nuts	1 cookie	230	27	16	4
Chocolate-White Chocolate Chunk	1 cookie	230	28	19	4¾
Oatmeal Raisin Pecan	1 cookie	220	29	18	4½
Peanut Butter Chocolate Chunk w/ Nuts	1 cookie	240	24	16	4
Peanut Butter w/ Nuts	1 cookie	240	24	15	3¾
Donuts					
Apple Crumb	1 donut	230	34	12	3
Bismark, Chocolate Iced	1 donut	340	50	31	7¾
Black Raspberry	1 donut	210	32	10	2½
Blueberry Cake Donut	1 donut	290	35	16	4

FOOD	SERVING SIZE	CALORIES	CARBO-HYDRATES (GRAMS)	SUGAR (GRAMS)	SUGAR (TSPS)
Donuts (continued)					
Blueberry Crumb Donut	1 donut	240	36	15	3¾
Boston Kreme Donut	1 donut	240	36	14	3½
Bow Tie Donut	1 donut	300	34	15	3¾
Butternut Cake Donut Ring	1 donut	300	36	16	4
Chocolate Cake Glazed Donut	1 donut	290	33	14	3½
Chocolate Coconut Cake Donut	1 donut	300	31	12	3
Chocolate Frosted Cake Donut	1 donut	300	38	18	4½
Chocolate Frosted Coffee Roll	1 donut	290	36	13	3¼
Chocolate Frosted Donut	1 donut	200	29	10	2½
Chocolate Kreme Filled Donut	1 donut	270	35	16	4
Cinnamon Cake Donut	1 donut	270	31	12	3
Coconut Cake Donut	1 donut	290	33	13	3¼
Coffee Roll	1 donut	270	33	10	2½
Double Chocolate Cake Donut	1 donut	310	37	18	4½
Éclair Donut	1 donut	270	39	17	4¼
Glazed Cake Donut	1 donut	270	33	14	3½
Glazed Chocolate Cruller	1 donut	280	36	16	4
Glazed Crullers	1 donut	290	37	18	4½
Jelly Filled Donut	1 donut	210	32	14	3½
Jelly Stick	1 donut	290	44	24	6
Lemon Donut	1 donut	200	28	8	2
Maple Frosted Coffee Roll	1 donut	290	36	13	3¼
Maple Frosted Donut	1 donut	210	30	12	3
Marble Frosted Donut	1 donut	200	29	11	2¾
Powdered Cake Donut	1 donut	270	32	13	3¼
Powdered Cruller	1 donut	270	30	11	2¾

FOOD	SERVING SIZE	CALORIES	CARBO-HYDRATES (GRAMS)	SUGAR (GRAMS)	SUGAR (TSPS)
Strawberry Donut	1 donut	210	32	11	2¾
Strawberry Frosted Donut	1 donut	210	30	12	3
Sugar Crullers	1 donut	250	27	8	2
Sugared Cake Donut	1 donut	250	27	9	2¼
Toasted Coconut Cake Donut	1 donut	300	35	16	4
Vanilla Frosted Coffee Roll	1 donut	290	36	13	3¼
Vanilla Frosted Donut	1 donut	210	30	12	3
Vanilla Kreme Filled Donut	1 donut	270	36	17	4¼
Whole wheat glazed cake donut	1 donut	310	32	14	3½

Drinks

FOOD	SERVING SIZE	CALORIES	CARBO-HYDRATES (GRAMS)	SUGAR (GRAMS)	SUGAR (TSPS)
Coffee Coolatta, all varieties	16 fl oz	230–410	51–52	50–51	12½–12¾
Dunkaccino	10 fl oz	250	34	24	6
Dunkaccino	14 fl oz	360	51	36	9
Dunkaccino	18 fl oz	480	67	48	12
Dunkaccino	20 fl oz	510	71	50	12½
Hot Cocoa	10 fl oz	230	38	29	7¼
Hot Cocoa	14 fl oz	330	57	43	10¾
Hot Cocoa	18 fl oz	440	75	57	14¼
Hot Cocoa	20 fl oz	470	79	61	15¼
Orange Mango Fruit Coolatta	16 fl oz	290	71	63	14¾
Pink Lemonade Fruit Coolatta	16 fl oz	350	88	63	15¾
Raspberry Lemonade Coolatta	16 fl oz	280	68	64	16
Strawberry Fruit Coolatta	16 fl oz	280	70	63	15¾
Vanilla Coolatta	16 fl oz	450	94	80	20

FOOD	SERVING SIZE	CALORIES	CARBO-HYDRATES (GRAMS)	SUGAR (GRAMS)	SUGAR (TSPS)
Munchkins					
Apple Cinnamon Pecan	1 munchkin	510	72	41	10¼
Apple & Spice	1 munchkin	350	57	29	7¼
Apple & Spice, low fat	1 munchkin	240	54	32	8
Banana, low fat	1 munchkin	250	57	35	8¾
Banana Nut	1 munchkin	360	52	29	7¼
Blueberry	1 4 oz munchkin	320	49	27	6¾
Blueberry	1 6 oz munchkin	490	76	41	10¼
Blueberry, low fat	1 munchkin	250	55	33	8¼
Blueberry, reduced fat	1 munchkin	450	77	42	10½
Bran	1 munchkin	390	60	34	8½
Bran, low fat	1 munchkin	240	57	32	8
Cherry	1 munchkin	340	53	29	7¼
Cherry, low fat	1 munchkin	250	56	34	8½
Chocolate, low fat	1 munchkin	250	53	29	7¼
Chocolate chip	1 4 oz munchkin	400	58	36	9
Chocolate chip	1 6 oz munchkin	590	88	50	12½
Chocolate Hazelnut Chunk	1 munchkin	610	87	52	13
Corn	1 4 oz munchkin	360	57	22	5½
Corn, low fat	1 munchkin	240	52	20	5
Corn, reduced fat	1 munchkin	460	79	35	8¾
Cranberry Orange	1 4 oz munchkin	470	76	41	10¼
Cranberry Orange	1 6 oz munchkin	240	55	32	8
Cranberry Orange Nut	1 munchkin	350	52	27	6¾
Honey Bran Raisin	1 munchkin	490	84	48	12
Lemon Poppyseed	1 munchkin	360	56	27	6¾
Oat Bran	1 munchkin	370	55	29	7¼

FOOD	SERVING SIZE	CALORIES	CARBO-HYDRATES (GRAMS)	SUGAR (GRAMS)	SUGAR (TSPS)

A Note about Dunkin' Donuts

Dunkin' Donuts Dunkaccinos are really loaded with sugar, but that's not all! These drinks and similar drinks also contain hydrogenated oils, chemicals, nonfat dry milk (more difficult to digest than regular milk), and coffee. Just look at this list of ingredients: sugar, nondairy creamer (contains partially hydrogenated soybean oil, corn syrup solids, sodium caseinate (a milk derivative), dipotassium phosphate, sugar, mono-and diglycerides, silicone dioxide, sodium steroyl lactylate, lecithin, artificial colors and artificial flavors, sweet cream (contains sweet cream, nonfat milk, sodium caseinate, lecithin, and bht), natural and artificial flavors, instant coffee, nonfat dry milk, cocoa powder (processed with alkali), cellulose gum, salt, and silicon dioxide. Think twice next time!

And, before you reach into that tempting box of donuts, be aware that not only do they have lots of sugar (Vanilla Kreme Filled contains sugar in six different forms), they also contain artificial colors and flavors, partially hydrogenated oils, preservatives, and other chemicals.

El Pollo Loco

FOOD	SERVING SIZE	CALORIES	CARBO-HYDRATES (GRAMS)	SUGAR (GRAMS)	SUGAR (TSPS)
Banana Split	1 serving	117	107	29	7¼
Berry Banana Smoothie	1 serving	367	68	27	6¾
Coleslaw	1 serving	206	12	5	1¼
Foster's Freeze (w/o cone)	1 serving	180	30	26	6½
Kiwi Strawberry Smoothie	1 serving	358	66	24	6
Smokey Black Bean Pollo Bowl	1 serving	604	75	20	5
Smokey Black Beans	1 serving	306	35	19	4¾

Foster's Freeze

See El Pollo Loco.

FOOD	SERVING SIZE	CALORIES	CARBO-HYDRATES (GRAMS)	SUGAR (GRAMS)	SUGAR (TSPS)

Häagen-Dazs

The ice cream listed below, which is served in the shops, is different from the ice cream that is sold at grocery stores.

Frozen Yogurt

FOOD	SERVING SIZE	CALORIES	CARBO-HYDRATES (GRAMS)	SUGAR (GRAMS)	SUGAR (TSPS)
Vanilla Fudge	½ cup	160	34	22	5½
Vanilla Raspberry Swirl	½ cup	130	29	20	5

Frozen Yogurt, Soft Serve, Nonfat

FOOD	SERVING SIZE	CALORIES	CARBO-HYDRATES (GRAMS)	SUGAR (GRAMS)	SUGAR (TSPS)
Coffee	½ cup	110	22	21	5¼
Chocolate	½ cup	110	23	20	5
Chocolate Mousse	½ cup	80	24	8	2
Strawberry	½ cup	110	24	23	5¾
Vanilla	½ cup	110	22	21	5¼
Vanilla Mousse	½ cup	70	23	8	2
White Chocolate	½ cup	110	22	21	5¼

Ice Cream

FOOD	SERVING SIZE	CALORIES	CARBO-HYDRATES (GRAMS)	SUGAR (GRAMS)	SUGAR (TSPS)
Baileys Irish Cream	½ cup	270	23	22	5½
Belgian Chocolate Chocolate	½ cup	320	29	26	6½
Brownies a la Mode	½ cup	280	28	23	5¾
Butter Pecan	½ cup	300	105	17	4¼
Cappuccino Commotion	½ cup	310	25	23	5¾
Chocolate	½ cup	260	21	20	5
Chocolate Chocolate Chip	½ cup	300	26	23	5¾
Chocolate Chocolate Mint	½ cup	300	25	22	5½
Chocolate Swiss Almond	½ cup	300	24	20	5
Coffee	½ cup	250	20	20	5

FOOD	SERVING SIZE	CALORIES	CARBO-HYDRATES (GRAMS)	SUGAR (GRAMS)	SUGAR (TSPS)
Ice Cream (continued)					
Coffee Fudge	½ cup	170	32	22	5½
Coffee Mocha Chip	½ cup	270	24	21	5¼
Cookie Dough Dynamo	½ cup	310	29	24	6
Cookies & Cream	½ cup	270	23	21	5¼
Cookies & Fudge	½ cup	180	33	20	5
Deep Chocolate Peanut Butter	½ cup	350	26	21	5¼
Dulce De Leche Caramel	½ cup	270	27	27	6¾
Macadamia Brittle	½ cup	280	24	23	5¾
Macadamia Nut	½ cup	320	20	19	4¾
Mint Chip	½ cup	280	25	22	5½
Pineapple Coconut	½ cup	230	25	24	6
Pistachio	½ cup	280	21	16	4
Pralines & Cream	½ cup	280	28	28	7
Rum Raisin	½ cup	260	21	20	5
Strawberry	½ cup	250	22	21	5¼
Vanilla	½ cup	250	20	20	5
Vanilla Chocolate Chip	½ cup	290	25	22	5½
Vanilla Swiss Almond	½ cup	290	23	20	5
Ice Cream Bars, Coated					
Chocolate & Dark Chocolate	½ cup	350	28	24	6
Coffee & Almond Crunch	½ cup	370	27	26	6½
Vanilla & Almonds	½ cup	380	26	24	6
Vanilla & Milk	½ cup	340	25	24	6
Ice Cream Bars, Uncoated					
Chocolate	½ cup	200	16	15	3¾

FOOD	SERVING SIZE	CALORIES	CARBO-HYDRATES (GRAMS)	SUGAR (GRAMS)	SUGAR (TSPS)
Ice Cream Bars, Uncoated (continued)					
Coffee	½ cup	190	15	15	3¾
Vanilla	½ cup	190	15	15	3¾
Sorbet					
Mango	½ cup	120	31	29	7¼
Orange	½ cup	120	30	24	6
Raspberry	½ cup	120	30	26	6½
Strawberry	½ cup	120	30	27	6¾
Zesty Lemon	½ cup	120	31	27	6¾
Sorbet, Soft Serve					
Raspberry	½ cup	110	28	25	6¼
Sorbet Bars					
Raspberry & Vanilla	½ cup	90	21	15	3¾

In-N-Out Burger

FOOD	SERVING SIZE	CALORIES	CARBO-HYDRATES (GRAMS)	SUGAR (GRAMS)	SUGAR (TSPS)
Burgers					
Hamburger	1 sandwich	390	39	10	2½
Cheeseburger	1 sandwich	480	39	10	2½
Double Double Cheeseburger	1 sandwich	670	40	10	2½
Drinks					
Chocolate Shake	15 fl oz	590	53	62	15½
Coca Cola Classic	16 fl oz	198	54	54	13½
Dr. Pepper	16 fl oz	200	52	52	13
Lemonade	16 fl oz	180	40	38	9½

FOOD	SERVING SIZE	CALORIES	CARBO-HYDRATES (GRAMS)	SUGAR (GRAMS)	SUGAR (TSPS)
Drinks (continued)					
Root Beer	16 fl oz	220	60	60	15
Seven Up	16 fl oz	220	52	52	13
Strawberry Shake	15 fl oz	690	104	96	24
Vanilla Shake	15 fl oz	580	78	57	14¼

Jack-in-the-Box

FOOD	SERVING SIZE	CALORIES	CARBO-HYDRATES (GRAMS)	SUGAR (GRAMS)	SUGAR (TSPS)
Breakfast					
French Toast Sticks w/ Bacon	16.3 oz	470	53	10	2½
Pancakes w/ Bacon	5.6 oz	370	59	14	3½
Syrup	1.0 oz	130	30	22	5½
Desserts					
Apple Pie	1 slice (3.5 oz)	370	54	28	7
Cheesecake	1 slice (3.8 oz)	320	32	22	5½
Double Fudge Cake	1 slice (10.6 oz)	300	50	25	6¼
Hot Apple Turnover	1 turnover (3.8 oz)	340	41	12	3
Drinks					
Barq's Rootbeer	20 fl oz	180	50	50	12½
Coca Cola Classic	20 fl oz	170	46	46	11½
Dr. Pepper	20 fl oz	190	53	53	13¾
Milk, reduced fat 2%	8 fl oz	130	14	14	3½
Minute Maid	20 fl oz	190	65	65	16¼
Orange Juice	10 fl oz	150	34	28	7
Sprite	20 fl oz	160	41	41	10¼

FOOD	SERVING SIZE	CALORIES	CARBO-HYDRATES (GRAMS)	SUGAR (GRAMS)	SUGAR (TSPS)
Ice Cream Shakes					
Cappuccino	16 fl oz	630	80	58	14½
Chocolate	16 fl oz	630	85	67	16¾
Oreo Cookie	16 fl oz	740	91	45	11¼
Strawberry	16 fl oz	640	85	67	16¾
Vanilla	16 fl oz	610	73	52	13
Sandwiches and Side Dishes					
Egg Rolls	5	730	67	9	2¼
Jack's Spicy Chicken	1	550	52	9	2¼
Jumbo Jack	2.4 oz	590	39	10	2½
Jumbo Jack w/ Cheese	10 oz	670	32	9	2¼
Sweet & Sour Dipping Sauce	1 packet	45	11	10	2½
Teriyaki Bowl	2.5 oz	670	128	27	6¾

Kentucky Fried Chicken

FOOD	SERVING SIZE	CALORIES	CARBO-HYDRATES (GRAMS)	SUGAR (GRAMS)	SUGAR (TSPS)
Chicken and Side Dishes					
BBQ Baked Beans	5.5 oz	190	33	13	3¼
Cole Slaw	5 oz	232	26	20	5
Chicken and Side Dishes					
Corn on the Cob	1 piece	150	35	8	2
Honey BBQ Wings	6 pieces	607	33	18	4½
Pot Pie	1 pie	770	69	8	2
Potato Salad	5.2 oz	230	23	9	2¼
Desserts					
Apple Pie Slice	4 oz	310	44	23	5¾
Chocolate Cream Pie	4 oz	290	37	25	6¼

FOOD	SERVING SIZE	CALORIES	CARBO-HYDRATES (GRAMS)	SUGAR (GRAMS)	SUGAR (TSPS)
Desserts (continued)					
Double Chocolate Chip Cake	2.7 oz	320	41	26	6½
Fudge Brownie	3.5 oz	280	44	35	8¾
Lemon Cream Pie	4.5 oz	410	62	50	12½
Little Bucket Parfaits, Chocolate Cream	4 oz	290	37	25	6¼
Little Bucket Parfaits, Fudge Brownie	3.5 oz	280	44	35	8¾
Little Bucket Parfaits, Lemon Creme	4.5 oz	410	62	50	12½
Little Bucket Parfaits, Strawberry Shortcake	3.5 oz	200	33	26	6½
Pecan Pie Slice	4 oz	490	66	31	7¾
Strawberry Creme Pie Slice	2.7 oz	280	32	22	5½
Strawberry Shortcake	3.5 oz	200	35	26	6½

Krispy Kreme Doughnuts

FOOD	SERVING SIZE	CALORIES	CARBO-HYDRATES (GRAMS)	SUGAR (GRAMS)	SUGAR (TSPS)
Cinnamon Apple Filled	1 doughnut	280	35	13	3¼
Fudge Iced Cake	1 doughnut	230	28	11	2¾
Fudge Iced Creme Filled	1 doughnut	340	39	22	5½
Fudge Iced Custard Filled	1 doughnut	310	39	21	5¼
Fudge Iced Glazed	1 doughnut	380	36	26	6½
Fudge Iced Glazed Cruller	1 doughnut	240	31	24	6
Fudge Iced Sprinkles	1 doughnut	220	31	19	4¾
Glazed Creme Filled	1 doughnut	350	39	24	6
Glazed Cruller	1 doughnut	250	24	15	3¾
Glazed Devil's Food	1 doughnut	390	41	30	7½
Glazed Lemon Filled	1 doughnut	280	33	15	3¾

FOOD	SERVING SIZE	CALORIES	CARBO-HYDRATES (GRAMS)	SUGAR (GRAMS)	SUGAR (TSPS)
Glazed Raspberry Filled	1 doughnut	270	37	20	5
Maple Iced Glazed	1 doughnut	200	28	18	4½
Original Glazed	1 doughnut	210	22	13	3¼

Mazzio's Pizza

Desserts

FOOD	SERVING SIZE	CALORIES	CARBO-HYDRATES (GRAMS)	SUGAR (GRAMS)	SUGAR (TSPS)
Cinnamon Sticks	4 pieces	350	45	12	3

Entrees

FOOD	SERVING SIZE	CALORIES	CARBO-HYDRATES (GRAMS)	SUGAR (GRAMS)	SUGAR (TSPS)
Fettuccine Alfredo	1 serving	1320	195	10	2½
Italian Sampler	1 serving	1640	206	15	3¾
Lasagna w/ meat sauce	1 serving	700	60	23	5¾
Spaghetti w/ marinara sauce	1 serving	940	208	20	5
Spaghetti w/ meat sauce, small	1 serving	1210	200	15	3¾
Spaghetti w/ meat sauce, medium	1 serving	1560	206	15	3¾
Pizzas have about ¾ tsp per 1 serving (⅛ of a pizza)					

McDonald's

Breakfast

FOOD	SERVING SIZE	CALORIES	CARBO-HYDRATES (GRAMS)	SUGAR (GRAMS)	SUGAR (TSPS)
Apple Danish	4 oz	360	51	29	7¼
Cheese Danish	4 oz	410	47	26	6½
Cinnamon Roll	3½ oz	390	50	24	6
Hotcakes, plain	5½ oz	340	58	14	3½
Hotcakes (w/ 2 pats margarine and syrup)	8 oz	610	104	45	11¼
Low-fat Apple Bran Muffin	4 oz	300	61	32	8

FOOD	SERVING SIZE	CALORIES	CARBO-HYDRATES (GRAMS)	SUGAR (GRAMS)	SUGAR (TSPS)
Desserts/Shakes					
Baked Apple Pie	2½ oz	260	34	13	3¼
Butterfinger McFlurry	12 fl oz	620	90	76	19
Chocolate Chip Cookie	1¼ oz	170	22	13	3¼
Chocolate Shake, small	14½ oz	360	60	54	13½
Hot Caramel Sundae	6½ oz	360	61	47	11¾
Hot Fudge Sundae	6½ oz	340	52	47	11¾
M & M McFlurry	12 fl oz	630	90	79	19¾
McDonaldland Cookies	1½ oz	180	32	12	3
Nestle Crunch McFlurry	12 fl oz	630	89	78	19½
Oreo McFlurry	12 fl oz	570	82	69	17¼
Strawberry shake, small	15 fl oz	360	60	55	13¾
Strawberry Sundae	6½ oz	290	50	46	11½
Vanilla Reduced Fat Ice Cream Cone	3 oz	150	23	17	4¼
Vanilla Shake, small	15 fl oz	360	59	55	13¾
Sandwiches					
Arch Deluxe	9 oz	550	39	8	2
Arch Deluxe with Bacon	9½ oz	590	39	8	2
Big Mac	8 oz	560	45	8	2
Quarter Pounder	6 oz	420	37	8	2
Quarter Pounder with Cheese	7 oz	530	38	9	2¼
Sauces and Salad Dressings					
Barbecue Sauce	1 pkg (1 oz)	45	10	10	2½
Fat-Free Herb Vinaigrette	1 pkg (2 oz)	50	11	9	2¼
Honey	1 pkg (½ oz)	45	12	11	2¾

FOOD	SERVING SIZE	CALORIES	CARBO-HYDRATES (GRAMS)	SUGAR (GRAMS)	SUGAR (TSPS)
Sauces and Salad					
Dressings (continued)					
Red French Reduced Calories	1 pkg (2 oz)	160	23	15	3¾
Sweet 'n Sour Sauce	1 pkg (1 oz)	50	11	10	2½
Soft Drinks/Milk/Juice					
1% Lowfat Milk	8 fl oz	100	13	13	3¼
Orange Juice	6 fl oz	80	20	18	4½
Coca-Cola Classic, child	12 fl oz	110	29	29	7¼
Coca-Cola, small	16 fl oz	150	40	40	10
Coca-Cola, med	21 fl oz	210	58	58	14½
Cola-Cola, large	32 fl oz	310	86	86	21½
Hi-C Orange Drink, child	12 fl oz	120	32	32	8
Hi-C Orange Drink, small	16 fl oz	160	44	44	11
Hi-C Orange Drink, med	21 fl oz	240	64	64	16
Hi-C Orange Drink, large	32 fl oz	350	94	94	23½
Sprite, child	12 fl oz	110	28	28	7
Sprite, small	16 fl oz	150	39	39	9¾
Sprite, med	21 fl oz	210	56	56	14
Sprite, large	32 fl oz	310	83	83	20¾

Panda Express

FOOD	SERVING SIZE	CALORIES	CARBO-HYDRATES (GRAMS)	SUGAR (GRAMS)	SUGAR (TSPS)
Chicken Orange	5 oz	310	31	18	4½
Sweet & Sour Sauce	2 oz	80	16	13	3¼

FOOD	SERVING SIZE	CALORIES	CARBO-HYDRATES (GRAMS)	SUGAR (GRAMS)	SUGAR (TSPS)
Popeyes					
Coleslaw	1 serving	233	20	15	3¾
Red Beans & Rice	1 serving	338	33	16	4
Pizza Hut					
Desserts					
Apple & Cherry Dessert Pizza	1 slice	250	48	25	6¼
Pasta					
Cavatini Pasta	1 serving	480	66	12	3
Cavatini Supreme	1 serving	560	72	11	2¾
Spaghetti w/ Marinara	1 serving	490	91	10	2½
Spaghetti w/ Meat Sauce	1 serving	600	98	10	2½
Spaghetti w/ Meatballs	1 serving	850	120	12	3
Pizza					
all pizzas	1 slice	279–376	45–48	8–9	2–2¼
Sandwich					
The Big New Yorker Cheese & Pepperoni	160–166	380–393	42	8	2
The Big New Yorker Supreme	210	459	44	15	3¾
Round Table Pizza					
Bacon Super Deli, Thin Crust	1 slice	200	16	15	3¾
Bacon Super Deli, Thick Crust	1 slice	260	26	25	6¼
Aloha Big Vinnie	1 slice	430	55	53	13¼
Big Vinnie	1 slice	460	49	46	11½

FOOD	SERVING SIZE	CALORIES	CARBO-HYDRATES (GRAMS)	SUGAR (GRAMS)	SUGAR (TSPS)
Cheese, Thin Crust	1 slice	160	16	15	3¾
Cheese, Thick Crust	1 slice	210	26	25	6¼
Chicken & Garlic Gourmet, Thin Crust	1 slice	170	17	16	4
Chicken & Garlic Gourmet, Thick Crust	1 slice	230	27	25	6¼
Classic Pesto, Thin Crust	1 slice	170	18	16	4
Classic Pesto, Thick Crust	1 slice	230	27	25	6¼
Garden Pesto, Thin Crust	1 slice	170	18	16	4
Garden Pesto, Thick Crust	1 slice	230	28	25	6¼
Gourmet Veggie Pizza, Thin Crust	1 slice	160	18	16	4
Gourmet Veggie Pizza, Thick Crust	1 slice	220	29	25	6¼
Guinevere's Garden Delight, Thin Crust	1 slice	150	18	16	4
Guinevere's Garden Delight, Thick Crust	1 slice	200	27	25	6¼
Italian Garlic Supreme, Thin Crust	1 slice	200	17	15	3¾
Italian Garlic Supreme, Thick Crust	1 slice	250	27	25	6¼
King Arthur's, Thin Crust	1 slice	200	18	15	3¾
King Arthur's, Thick Crust	1 slice	240	27	25	6¼
Maui Zaui, Thin Crust	1 slice	170	18	17	4¼
Maui Zaui, Thick Crust	1 slice	310	37	35	8¾
Pepperoni, Thin Crust	1 slice	170	17	15	3¾
Pepperoni, Thick Crust	1 slice	220	26	25	6¼
Saute Chicken & Garlic, Thin Crust	1 slice	150	18	16	4

FOOD	SERVING SIZE	CALORIES	CARBO-HYDRATES (GRAMS)	SUGAR (GRAMS)	SUGAR (TSPS)
Saute Chicken & Garlic, Thick Crust	1 slice	200	28	25	6¼
Saute Veggie, Thin Crust	1 slice	140	19	16	4
Saute Veggie, Thick Crust	1 slice	190	28	25	6¼
Western BBQ Chicken Supreme, Thin Crust	1 slice	170	25	18	4½
Western BBQ Chicken Supreme, Thick Crust	1 slice	220	30	27	6¾

Schlotzsky's

Sandwiches

FOOD	SERVING SIZE	CALORIES	CARBO-HYDRATES (GRAMS)	SUGAR (GRAMS)	SUGAR (TSPS)
Albacore Tuna, large	1 sandwich	1000	147	11	2¾
Albacore Tuna Melt, large	1 sandwich	1631	158	14	3½
Cheese Original, large	1 sandwich	1857	159	13	3¼
Chicken Breast, large	1 sandwich	1008	158	12	3
Chicken Club, large	1 sandwich	1351	149	11	2¾
Corned Beef, large	1 sandwich	1134	139	13	3¼
Deluxe Original, large	1 sandwich	2638	173	28	7
Dijon Chicken, large	1 sandwich	972	150	11	2¾
Ham & Cheese Original, med	1 sandwich	1625	161	18	4½
Ham & Cheese Original, large	1 sandwich	1917	166	22	5½
Pastrami & Swiss, large	1 sandwich	1681	148	13	3¼
Pastrami Reuben, large	1 sandwich	1777	152	15	3¾
Pesto Chicken, large	1 sandwich	999	147	10	2½
Philly, large	1 sandwich	1709	157	12	3
Roast Beef, large	1 sandwich	816	79	9	2¼
Roast Beef & Cheese, large	1 sandwich	1749	163	13	3¼
Santa Fe Chicken, large	1 sandwich	1182	169	17	4¼

FOOD	SERVING SIZE	CALORIES	CARBO-HYDRATES (GRAMS)	SUGAR (GRAMS)	SUGAR (TSPS)
Sandwiches (continued)					
Smoked Turkey Breast, large	1 sandwich	988	150	12	3
Texas Schlotzskys, large	1 sandwich	1544	155	18	4½
Texas Schlotzskys, large	1 sandwich	2083	166	18	4½
Turkey & Bacon Club	1 sandwich	1790	161	14	3½
Turkey Guacamole, large	1 sandwich	1317	166	17	4¼
Turkey Reuben, large	1 sandwich	1656	159	12	3
Vegetable Club, large	1 sandwich	1112	51	11	2¾
Vegetarian, large	1 sandwich	966	150	14	3½
Western Vegetarian, large	1 sandwich	1261	150	13	3¼
Sides					
Coleslaw, all varieties	1 side	225	16	16	4
Potato Salad, Diced w/ Egg	1 side	216	18	10	2½
Vegetable Cheese Soup	1 side	289	24	11	2¾

Subway

FOOD	SERVING SIZE	CALORIES	CARBO-HYDRATES (GRAMS)	SUGAR (GRAMS)	SUGAR (TSPS)
Desserts					
Brazil Nut Cookie	1 cookie	214	29	17	4¼
Chocolate Chip M & M Cookie	1 cookie	212	29	17	4¼
Oatmeal Raisin	1 cookie	199	29	17	4¼
Oatmeal Raisin, low fat	1 cookie	168	33	18	4½

Sandwiches

All varieties of sandwiches have approximately two to two and a half teaspoons of sugar.

FOOD	SERVING SIZE	CALORIES	CARBO-HYDRATES (GRAMS)	SUGAR (GRAMS)	SUGAR (TSPS)
Taco Bell					
Taco Salads					
Taco Salad w/ Salsa	19 oz	850	69	12	3
Taco Salad w/ Salsa w/o Shell	16½ oz	435	36	12	3
Drinks					
Dr Pepper	16 fl oz	208	62	62	15½
Lipton Brisk Iced Tea Sweetened	16 fl oz	140	40	40	10
Mountain Dew	16 fl oz	227	61	61	15¼
Orange Juice	6 fl oz	80	18	18	4½
Pepsi-Cola	16 fl oz	200	55	55	13¾
Reduced Fat Milk	8 fl oz	110	11	10	2½
Slice	16 fl oz	200	53	52	13
Desserts					
Choco Taco Ice Cream Dessert	1 serving	310	37	27	6¾
Cinnamon Twist	1 twist	180	25	10	2½
Taco John's					
Desserts					
Apple Grande	1 grande	258	40	14	3½
Choco Taco	1 taco	311	37	27	6¼
Cinnamon Mint Swirl	1 piece	60	14	14	3½
Dichos Cookies	3 cookies	100	33	10	2½
Salads					
Chicken Fajita Salad	1 salad	646	53	9	2¼
Taco Salad	1 salad	716	55	8	2

FOOD	SERVING SIZE	CALORIES	CARBO-HYDRATES (GRAMS)	SUGAR (GRAMS)	SUGAR (TSPS)
TCBY					
Lowfat Ice Cream, all flavors	½ cup	120	22	18	4½
96% Fat-Free Frozen Yogurt, all flavors	½ cup	130	23	20	5
Nonfat Soft-Serve Frozen Yogurt, all flavors	½ cup	110	23	20	5
Sorbet, all flavors	½ cup	100	24	19	4¾
Treatzza Pizza & Cake					
Health Treatzza Pizza	⅛ pie (2.3 oz)	180	28	18	4½
M&M's Treatzza Pizza	⅛ pie (2.5 oz)	190	29	20	5
Round Cake, frozen 8"	⅛ cake (6.5 oz)	370	56	42	10½
Round Cake, layered 8"	⅛ cake (5.25 oz)	330	49	39	9¾
Wendy's					
Breakfast					
French Toast Sticks with Bacon	4.7 oz	470	53	10	2½
Syrup	1.5 oz	130	30	22	5½
Desserts					
Carrot Cake	1 piece (3.5 oz)	370	54	28	7
Cheesecake	1 piece (3.7 oz)	320	32	22	5½
Chocolate Chip Cookie	1 cookie	270	36	16	4
Double Fudge Cake	1 piece (3 oz)	300	50	25	6¼
Frosty Dairy Dessert, small	12 fl oz	340	91	47	11¾
Frosty Dairy Dessert, med	16 fl oz	460	56	43	10¾
Frosty Dairy Dessert, large	20 fl oz	570	91	79	19¾
Hot Apple Turnover	1 piece (3.8 oz)	340	41	12	3

FOOD	SERVING SIZE	CALORIES	CARBO-HYDRATES (GRAMS)	SUGAR (GRAMS)	SUGAR (TSPS)
Drinks					
Barq's Root Beer	20 fl oz	180	50	50	12½
Coca Cola Classic	20 fl oz	170	46	46	11½
Dr Pepper	20 fl oz	190	53	53	13¼
Hi-C Orange Drink, small	16 fl oz	160	44	44	11
Hi-C Orange Drink, med	21 fl oz	240	64	64	16
Hi-C Orange Drink, large	32 fl oz	350	94	94	23½
Orange Juice	10 fl oz	150	34	28	7
Minute Maid Lemonade	20 fl oz	190	65	65	16¼
Sprite	20 fl oz	160	41	41	10¼
Ice Cream Shakes					
Cappuccino	16 fl oz	630	80	58	14¼
Chocolate	16 fl oz	630	85	67	16¾
Oreo Cookie	16 fl oz	740	91	45	11¼
Strawberry	16 fl oz	640	85	67	16¾
Vanilla	16 fl oz	610	73	65	16¼
Sandwiches, Salads, and Side Dishes					
Baked Potato, all varieties	1 potato	380–570	74–80	7–9	1¾–2¼
Chicken Sandwich, grilled	1 sandwich	310	35	8	2
Chicken Sandwiches, all other varieties	1 sandwich	410–490	43–44	7–8	1¾–2
Chicken Teriyaki Bowl	17.9 oz	570	128	27	6¾
Chili, large	12 oz	310	32	8	2
Egg Rolls	5 rolls	730	67	9	2¼
Garden Veggie Pita	1 pita	430	52	8	2

FOOD	SERVING SIZE	CALORIES	CARBO-HYDRATES (GRAMS)	SUGAR (GRAMS)	SUGAR (TSPS)
Sandwiches, Salads, and Side Dishes (continued)					
Hamburger & Cheeseburgers, all varieties	3.9–9.9 oz	270–570	30–37	7–11	1¾–2¾
Jack's Spicy Chicken	8.9 oz	570	52	9	2¼
Taco Salad	1 salad	390	28	9	2¼
Sauces and Dressing					
Chicken Nugget Sauce, Honey	1 oz	130	5	5	1¼
Sweet & Sour Sauce	1 oz	28	11	10	2½
Thousand Island Dressing	2 oz	250	10	8	2

White Castle

FOOD	SERVING SIZE	CALORIES	CARBO-HYDRATES (GRAMS)	SUGAR (GRAMS)	SUGAR (TSPS)
Chocolate Shake	1	310	46	39	9¾
Vanilla Shake	1	310	37	27	6¾

Yoplait and Colombo

FOOD	SERVING SIZE	CALORIES	CARBO-HYDRATES (GRAMS)	SUGAR (GRAMS)	SUGAR (TSPS)
Yoplait					
99% Fat-Free Strawberry	8 oz	230	43	35	8¾
Nonfat Plain	6 oz	100	14	10	2½
Colombo					
Fruit Flavors, low fat	8 oz	200	36	33	8¼
Plain, low fat	8 oz	130	12	11	2¾
Strawberry, low fat	8 oz	180	27	25	6¼
Vanilla, low fat	8 oz	180	29	28	7

Sources for "110 Reasons Why Sugar Is Ruining Your Health"

1. Sanchez, A., et al. "Role of Sugars in Human Neutrophilic Phagocytosis," *American Journal of Clinical Nutrition* 261 (November 1973): 1180–1184.
2. Couzy, F., et al. "Nutritional Implications of the Interaction Minerals," *Progressive Food and Nutrition Science* 17 (1933): 65–87.
3. Goldman, J., et al. "Behavioral Effects of Sucrose on Preschool Children," *Journal of Abnormal Child Psychology* 14, No. 4 (1986): 565–577.
4. Scanto, S. and Yudkin, J. "The Effect of Dietary Sucrose on Blood Lipids, Serum Insulin, Platelet Adhesiveness and Body Weight in Human Volunteers," *Postgraduate Medicine Journal* 45 (1969): 602–607.
5. Ringsdorf, W., Cheraskin, E. and Ramsay R. "Sucrose Neutrophilic Phagocytosis and Resistance to Disease," *Dental Survey*, 52, No. 12 (1976): 46–48.
6. Cerami, A., Vlassara, H., and Brownlee, M. "Glucose and Aging," *Scientific American* (May 1987): 90.
7. Albrink, M. and Ullrich I. H. "Interaction of Dietary

Sucrose and Fiber on Serum Lipids in Healthy Young Men Fed High Carbohydrate Diets," *American Journal of Clinical Nutrition* 43 (1986): 419–428.

8. Kozlovsky, A., et al. "Effects of Diets High in Simple Sugars on Urinary Chromium Losses," *Metabolism* 35 (June 1986): 515–518.
9. Takahashi, E., Tohoku University School of Medicine, *Wholistic Health Digest* (October 1982) 41.
10. Kelsay, J., et al. "Diets High in Glucose or Sucrose and Young Women," *American Journal of Clinical Nutrition* 27 (1974): 926–936.
11. Fields, M., et al. "Effect of Copper Deficiency on Metabolism and Mortality in Rats Fed Sucrose or Starch Diets," *Journal of Clinical Nutrition* 113 (1983): 1335–1345.
12. Lemann, J. "Evidence that Glucose Ingestion Inhibits Net Renal Tubular Reabsorption of Calcium and Magnesium," *Journal of Clinical Nutrition* 70 (1967): 236–245.
13. Taub, H. Ed. "Sugar Weakens Eyesight," *VM Newsletter* 5 (May, 1986).
14. "Sugar, White Flour Withdrawal Produces Chemical Response," *The Addiction Letter* (July 1992): 4.
15. Dufty, William. *Sugar Blues*. New York: Warner Books, 1975.
16. Ibid.
17. Jones, T. W., et al. "Enhanced Adrenomedullary Response and Increased Susceptibility to Neuroglygopenia: Mechanisms Underlying the Adverse Effect of Sugar Ingestion on Children," *Journal of Pediatrics* 126 (2) (Feb. 1995): 171–7.

18. Ibid.
19. Lee, A. T. and Cerami A. "The Role of Glycation in Aging," *Annals of the New York Academy of Science* 663 (1992): 63–70.
20. Abrahamson, E. and Peget A. *Body, Mind and Sugar.* New York: Avon, 1977.
21. Glinsmann, W., Irausquin, H., and Youngmee, K. "Evaluation of Health Aspects of Sugar Contained in Carbohydrate Sweeteners." *F.D.A. Report of Sugars Task Force.* (1986): 39.

    Makinen K. K., et al. "A Descriptive Report of the Effects of a 16–month Xylitol Chewing-gum Programme Subsequent to a 40–month Sucrose Gum Programme," *Caries Research* 32(2) (1998):107–12.
22. Keen, H., et al. "Nutrient Intake, Adiposity, and Diabetes," *British Medical Journal,* 1 (1989):655–658.
23. Yudkin, J. *Sweet and Dangerous.* New York: Bantam Books, (1974): 129.
24. Ibid.
25. Darlington, L., Ramsey, N. W. and Mansfield, J. R. "Placebo-Controlled, Blind Study of Dietary Manipulation Therapy in Rheumatoid Arthritis," *Lancet* 1: 8475 (Feb. 1, 1986):236–238.
26. Powers, L. "Sensitivity: You React to What You Eat," *Los Angeles Times* (Feb. 12, 1985).
27. Crook, W. *The Yeast Connection.* Jackson, TN: Professional Books, 1984.
28. Heaton, K. "The Sweet Road to Gallstones," *British Medical Journal* 288 (April 14, 1984): 1103–4.

    Misciagna, G., et al. *American Journal of Clinical Nutrition* 69 (1999): 120–126.

29. Yudkin, J. "Dietary Fat and Dietary Sugar in Relation to Ischemic Heart Disease and Diabetes," *Lancet* 2: No. 4.

Suadicani, P., et al. "Adverse Effects of Risk of Ishaemic Heart Disease of Adding Sugar to Hot Beverages in Hypertensives Using Diuretics," *Blood Pressure* 5, No. 2 (Mar 1996): 71–91.

30. Cleave, T. *The Saccharine Disease.* New Canaan, CT: Keats Publishing, 1974.

31. Erlander, S. "The Cause and Cure of Multiple Sclerosis," *The Disease to End Disease,* 1, No.3 (March 3, 1979): 59–63

32. Cleave, T. *The Saccharine Disease.* New Canaan, CT: Keats Publishing, 1974.

33. Cleave, T. and Campbell, G. *Diabetes, Coronary Thrombosis and the Saccharine Disease.* Bristol, England: John Wright and Sons, 1960.

34. Behall, K. "Influence of Estrogen Content of Oral Contraceptives and Consumption of Sucrose on Blood Parameters," *Disease Abstracts International* 43 (1982): 1437.

35. Glinsmann, W., Irausquin, H., and K. Youngmee. *Evaluation of Health Aspects of Sugar Contained in Carbohydrate Sweeteners.* F.D.A. Report of Sugars Task Force. (1986) 36–39.

36. TjSderhane, L. and Larmas , M. "A High Sucrose Diet Decreases the Mechanical Strength of Bones in Growing Rats," *Journal of Nurition* 128 (1998): 1807–1810.

37. Appleton, N. *Healthy Bones.* Garden City Park, New York: Avery Publishing, 1989; 19.

38. Beck-Nielsen H., Pedersen O., and Schwartz S. "Ef-

fects of Diet on the Cellular Insulin binding and the Insulin Sensitivity in Young Healthy Subjects," *Diabetes* 15 (1978): 289–296.

39. Thomas, B. J., et al. "Relation of Habitual Diet to Fasting Plasma Insulin Concentration and the Insulin Response to Oral Glucose," *Human Nutrition Clinical Nutrition* 36C, No. 1 (1982): 49–51.
40. Gardner, L., and Reiser, S. "Effects Dietary Carbohydrate on Fasting Levels of Human Growth Hormone and Cortisol," *Proceedings of the Society for Experimental Biology and Medicine* 169 (1982): 36–40.
41. Reiser, S. "Effects of Dietary Sugars on Metabolic Risk Factors Associated with Heart Disease," *Nutritional Health* 3 (1985): 203–216.
42. Hodges, R., and Rebello, T. "Carbohydrates and Blood Pressure," *Annals of Internal Medicine* 98 (1983): 838–841.
43. Behar, D., et al. "Sugar Challenge Testing with Children Considered Behaviorally Sugar Reactive," *Nutritional Behavior* 1 (1984): 277–288.
44. Grand, E. "Food Allergies and Migraine," *Lancet* 1 (1979): 955–959.
45. Simmons, J. "Is the Sand of Time Sugar?" *Longevity* (June 1990): 49–53.
46. Appleton, Nancy. *Lick the Sugar Habit*. Garden City Park, New York: Avery Publishing Group, 1988.
47. "Sucrose Induces Diabetes in Cat," *Federal Protocol* 6, No. 97 (1974).
48. Cleave, T. *The Saccharine Disease*. New Canaan, CT: Keats Publishing, Inc., 1974; 131.
49. Ibid., p 132.

50. Vaccaro O, Ruth K. J., and Stamler J. "Relationship of Postload Plasma Glucose to Mortality with 19–yr Follow-up." *Diabetes Care* 10 (Oct. 15, 1992):1328–34. Tominaga, M., et al., "Impaired Glucose Tolerance Is a Risk Factor for Cardiovascular Disease, but Not Fasting Glucose," *Diabetes Care* 22, No. 6 (1999): 920–924.
51. Lee, A. T. and Cerami, A. "Modifications of Proteins and Nucleic Acids by Reducing Sugars: Possible Role in Aging," *Handbook of the Biology of Aging*. New York: Academic Press, 1990.
52. Monnier, V. M. "Nonenzymatic Glycosylation, the Maillard Reaction and the Aging Process," *Journal of Gerontology*, 45, No. 4 (1990): 105–110.
53. Dyer, D. G., et al. "Accumulation of Maillard Reaction Products in Skin Collagen in Diabetes and Aging," *Journal of Clinical Investigation* 91, No. 6 (June 1993): 421–22.
54. Rattan, S. I., et al. "Protein Synthesis, Post-translational Modifications, and Aging." *Annals of the New York Academy of Sciences* 663 (1992): 48–62.
55. Monnier, V. M. "Nonenzymatic Glycosylation, the Maillard Reaction and the Aging Process," *Journal of Gerontology*, 45, No. 4 (1990): 105–110.
56. Pamplona, R., et al. "Mechanisms of Glycation in Atherogenesis," *Medical Hypotheses* 40 (1990): 174–181.
57. Ibid.
58. Ibid.
59. Appleton, Nancy. *Lick the Sugar Habit*. Garden City Park, New York: Avery Publishing Group, 1988.
60. Cerami, A., Vlassara, H., and Brownlee, M. "Glucose and Aging," *Scientific American* (May 1987): 90.

61. Goulart, F. S. "Are You Sugar Smart?" *American Fitness* (March–April 1991): 34–38.
62. Ibid.
63. Yudkin, J., Kang, S. and Bruckdorfer, K. "Effects of High Dietary Sugar," *British Journal of Medicine* 281 (November 22, 1980):1396.
64. Goulart, F. S. "Are You Sugar Smart?" *American Fitness* (March–April 1991): 34–38.
65. Ibid.
66. Ibid.
67. Ibid.
68. Ibid.
69. Nash, J. "Health Contenders," *Essence* 23 (January 1992) 79–81. As told by Elsie Morris, M.D., of Atlanta, a specialist in allergy and immunology.
70. Greenberg, Kurt. Interviewed John P. Trowbridge, M.D., "An Update on the Yeast Connection," *Health News and Review* (Spring, 1990) 10.
71. Goulart F. S. "Are You Sugar Smart?" *American Fitness* (March–April 1991): 34–38.
72. Schauss, A. *Diet, Crime and Delinquency.* Berkeley CA: Parker House, 1981.
73. Christensen, L. "The Role of Caffeine and Sugar in Depression," *The Nutrition Report* 9, No. 3 (March 1991): 17, 24.
74. Ibid.
75. Cornee, J., et al. "A Case-control Study of Gastric Cancer and Nutritional Factors in Marseille, France," *European Journal of Epidemiology* 11 (1995): 55–65.
76. Yudkin, J. *Sweet and Dangerous.* New York: Bantam Books, (1974): 129.

77. Ibid, 44.
78. Reiser, S., et al. "Effects of Sugars on Indices on Glucose Tolerance in Humans," *American Journal of Clinical Nutrition* 43 (1986): 151–159.
79. Ibid.
80. Kruis, W., et al. "Effects of Diets Low and High in Refined Sugars on Gut Transit, Bile Acid Metabolism and Bacterial Fermentation," *Gut* 32 (1991): 367–370.
81. Monnier, V., "Nonenzymatic Glycosylation, the Maillard Reaction and the Aging Process," *Journal of Gerontology* 45, No. 4 (1990) B105–111.
82. Persson P. G., Ahlbom, A., and Hellers, G. *Epidemiology* 3, No. 1 (1992): 47–52.
83. Yudkin, J. "Metabolic Changes Induced by Sugar in Relation to Coronary Heart Disease and Diabetes," *Nutrition and Health* 5, No. 1–2 (1987): 5–8.
84. Ibid.
85. Curhan, G., et al. "Beverage Use and Risk for Kidney Stones in Women," *Annals of Internal Medicine*, 1998, 128: 534–540.
86. *Journal of Advanced Medicine*, 7, No.1 (1994): 51–58.
87. Ibid.
88. Ibid.
89. *Postgraduate Medicine*, Sept 1969: 45 No. 527:602–07.
90. Moerman, C. J., et al. "Dietary Sugar Intake in the Etiology of Biliary Tract Cancer," *International Journal of Epidemiology* 22, No.2 (April 1993):207–214.
91. Ibid.
92. Lenders, C. M., "Gestational Age and Infant Size at Birth Are Associated with Dietary Intake Among Preg-

nant Adolescents," *Journal of Nutrition* 127 (June 1997): 1,113–1,117.

93. Ibid.
94. R. M. Bostick,R. M., et al. "Sugar, Meat and Fat Intake, and Non-Dietary risk factors for Colon Cancer Incidence in Iowa Women," *Cancer Causes Control* 5 (1994): 38–53.
95. Ibid.

    Ludwig, D. S., et al. "High Glycemic Index Foods, Overeating and Obesity," *Pediatrics* 103, No. 3 (March 1999): 26–32.
96. Hallfrisch, J., et al. "Effects of Dietary Fructose on Plasma Glucose and Hormone Responses in Normal and Hyperinsulinemic Men," *Journal of Nutrition* 113, No. 9 (Sept. 1983): 1,819–1,826.
97. Lee, A. T. and Cerami A. "The Role of Glycation in Aging," *Annals of the New York Academy of Science* 663 (1992): 63–70.
98. Moerman, C., et al. "Dietary Sugar Intake in the Etiology of Biliary Tract Cancer," *International Journal of Epidemiology* 22, No. 2 (April 1993):207–214.
99. "Sugar, White Flour Withdrawal Produces Chemical Response," *The Addiction Letter* (July 1992):4.
100. Ibid.
101. *The Edell Health Letter* 10, No.7 (Sept 1991) 1.
102. Bernstein, J., et al. "Depression of Lymphosyte Transformation Following Oral Glucose Ingestion," *American Journal of Clinical Nutrition* 30 (1977): 613.
103. Christensen L., Krietsch K., White B. and Stagner B. "Impact of a Dietary Change on Emotional Distress,"

Journal of Abnormal Psychology 94, No. 4 (1985):565–79.

104. *Nutrition Health Review*, Fall 1985.
105. Ludwig, D. S., et al. "High Glycemic Index Foods, Overeating and Obesity," *Pediatrics* 103, No. 3 (March 1999): 26–32.
106. *Pediatrics Research* 38, No. 4 (1995): 539–542.
107. Blacklock, N. J. "Sucrose and Idiopathic Renal Stone," *Nutrition Health*, 5, No. 1 & 2 (1987):9–17.
108. Lechin, F., et al. "Effects of an Oral Glucose Load on Plasma Neurotransmitters in Humans," *Neurophychobiology* 26, No. 1–2 (1992): 4–11.
109. Fields, M. *Journal of the American College of Nutrition* 17, No. 4 (August, 1998): 317–21.
110. De Stefani, E. "Dietary Sugar and Lung Cancer: a Case-control Study in Uruguay," *Nutrition and Cancer* 31, No. 2 (1998):132–7.

References

Published Material

Composition of Foods, Raw, Processed, Prepared. U.S. Dept. of Agriculture, Human Nutrition Information Service. Washington, D.C.: U.S. Government Printing Office. 1976 1992.

Gebhardt, Susan E. and Matthews, Ruth H. *Home and Garden Bulletin Number* 72, United States Department of Agriculture, Superintendent of Documents, U.S. Government Printing Office, Washington D.C. 20402, 1992.

Hands, Elizabeth S., *Nutrients in Foods*. Philadelphia, PA: Lippincott, Williams & Wilkins, 2000.

Jacobson, Michael and Sarah Frischner. *The Fast-Food Guide*, 2nd edition, New York, NY: Workman Publications, 1991.

Mathews, Ruth H., Pehrsson, Pamela R. and Mojgan Farhat-Sabet. Home Economics Research Report No. 48, 1987. *Sugar Content of Selected Foods: Individual and Total Sugars*. U.S. Department of Agriculture.

Natow, Annette B. and Heslin, Jo Ann. *The Carbohydrate, Fiber, and Sugar Counter*. New York: Pocket Books, 1999.

Pennington, Jean A. T. *Food Values of Portions Commonly Used*, 17th edition, Philadelphia, PA: Lippincott, 1998.

Internet Home Pages

Fast food information on line:

www.henkuhl.com/fastfoods
www.nutribase.com

Grocery stores on line:

www.albertson.com (for access use 98001 for the zip code)
www.groceronline.com
www.homerunners.com (for access use 02116 for the zip code)
www.netgrocer.com
www.webvan.com

Nutrition/Medical Information on line:

www.mercola.com
www.price-pottenger.org